Medical Ethics: A Very Short Introduction

VERY SHORT INTRODUCTIONS are for anyone wanting a stimulating and accessible way into a new subject. They are written by experts, and have been translated into more than 45 different languages.

The series began in 1995, and now covers a wide variety of topics in every discipline. The VSI library now contains over 500 volumes—a Very Short Introduction to everything from Psychology and Philosophy of Science to American History and Relativity—and continues to grow in every subject area.

Titles in the series include the following:

Tony Hope

MEDICAL ETHICS

A Very Short Introduction

OXFORD
UNIVERSITY PRESS

Great Clarendon Street, Oxford OX2 6DP

Oxford University Press is a department of the University of Oxford.
It furthers the University's objective of excellence in research, scholarship,
and education by publishing worldwide in

Oxford New York

Auckland Bangkok Buenos Aires Cape Town Chennai
Dar es Salaam Delhi Hong Kong Istanbul Karachi Kolkata
Kuala Lumpur Madrid Melbourne Mexico City Mumbai Nairobi
São Paulo Shanghai Taipei Tokyo Toronto

Oxford is a registered trade mark of Oxford University Press
in the UK and in certain other countries

Published in the United States
by Oxford University Press Inc., New York

British Library Cataloguing in Publication Data
Data available

Library of Congress Cataloging in Publication Data
Data available
ISBN 978-0-19-280282-8

19 20

Typeset by RefineCatch Ltd, Bungay, Suffolk
Printed in Great Britain by
Ashford Colour Press Ltd, Gosport, Hants.

This book is dedicated to my parents, Marion and Ronald Hope, who inspired my love of reading and reasoning.

LORD FOPPINGTON: Why, that's the fatigue I speak of, madam. For 'tis impossible to be quiet, without thinking: now thinking is to me the greatest fatigue in the world.

AMANDA: Does not your lordship love reading then?

LORD FOPPINGTON: Oh, passionately, madam. – But I never think of what I read.

BERINTHIA: Why, how can your lordship read without thinking?

LORD FOPPINGTON: O Lard! – can your ladyship pray without devotion, madam?

AMANDA: Well, I must own I think books the best entertainment in the world.

LORD FOPPINGTON: I am so very much of your ladyship's mind, madam, that I have a private gallery (where I walk sometimes) is furnished with nothing but books and looking glasses. Madam, I have gilded 'em, and ranged 'em so prettily, before Gad, it is the most entertaining thing in the world to walk and look upon 'em.

AMANDA: Nay, I love a neat library, too; but 'tis, I think, the inside of the book should recommend it most to us.

LORD FOPPINGTON: That, I must confess, I am nat altogether so fand of. Far to mind the inside of a book, is to entertain one's self with the forced product of another man's brain.

(John Vanbrugh, *The Relapse*, Act II, scene I)

Acknowledgements

I would like to thank the following. M. T. V. Hart who introduced me to philosophy; Jonathan Glover, whose philosophy tutorials are amongst the most stimulating intellectual experiences in my life; Mike Gaze who supervised my Ph.D. and who showed me how experimental science and theoretical ideas could work together in creative tension; Rosamond Rhodes, Stefan Baumrin, and their colleagues at Mount Sinai Medical School in New York whose annual conference provided a critical but supportive forum for developing several of the ideas in this book; Arthur Kuflik, whose incisive comments, at all levels, on the draft manuscript helped me make many improvements; Caroline Miles for her unstinting, imaginative and skilful support in developing practical medical ethics in Oxford.

I have been stimulated and educated by discussions with many colleagues and friends, including: Julian Savulescu, Mike Parker, John McMillan, Guy Widdershoven, Roger Crisp, Martyn Evans, Bill Fulford, Don Hill, Andreas Hasman, Anne Slowther, Jacinta Tan, Clive Baldwin, Ranaan Gillon, Ken Boyd, Tom Murray, Murray Longmore, Richard Ashcroft, Theo Schofield, Sarah Ford, Catherine Hood, Iain Chalmers.

I would like to thank all those at Oxford University Press who have helped to make this book possible and who have given their support and advice, including Shelley Cox; Emma Simmons, Debbie Protheroe,

Marsha Fillion, and Alison Langton; and Peter Butcher of RefineCatch Limited.

Finally I would like to thank my wife, Sally, and daughters Katy and Beth for their support, detailed discussions, and inspiration.

Contents

List of illustrations

The publisher and the author apologize for any errors or omissions in the above list. If contacted they will be pleased to rectify these at the earliest opportunity.

Chapter 1
On why medical ethics is exciting

'I don't have a lot of time for thinking about things' he said with a
defensive edge creeping into his tone. 'I just scatter my hundreds
and thousands before the public. Philosophy I leave to the drunks.'

(Ice-cream stall owner, in Malcom Pryce,
Aberystwyth Mon Amour)

Medical ethics will appeal to many temperaments: to the thinker
and to the doer; to the philosopher and to the woman or man
of action. It deals with some of the big moral questions: easing
death and the morality of killing, for example. It takes us into the
realm of political philosophy. How should health care resources,
necessarily limited, be distributed, and what should be the process
for deciding? It is concerned with legal issues. Should it always be a
crime for a doctor to practise euthanasia? When can a mentally ill
person be treated against his will? And it leads us to the major
world issue of the proper relationships between rich and poor
countries.

Modern medical science creates new moral choices, and challenges
traditional views that we have of ourselves. Cloning has inspired
many films and much concern. The possibility of making creatures
that are part human and part from some other animal is not far off.
Reproductive technologies raise the apparently abstract question of
how we should think about the interests of those who are yet to be

born – and who may never exist. This question leads us beyond medicine to consider our responsibilities towards the future of mankind.

Medical ethics ranges from the metaphysical to the mundanely practical. It is concerned not only with these large issues but also with everyday medical practice. Doctors get caught up in people's lives, and ordinary life is full of ethical tensions. An elderly woman with a degree of dementia suffers an acute life-threatening illness. Should she be treated in hospital with all the drugs and technology available; or should she be kept comfortable at home? The family cannot agree. There is nothing in this case likely to hit the headlines; but, as Auden's Old Masters knew, the ordinary is what is important to most of us, most of the time. In pursuing medical ethics we must be prepared to grapple with theory, allowing time for speculation and the use of the imagination. But we must also be ready to be practical: able to adopt a no-nonsense, down-to-earth, approach.

My own interest in medical ethics started at the theoretical end of the spectrum when studying for a degree that included philosophy. But when I went to medical school my inclination turned more to the practical. Decisions had to be made, and sick people had to be helped. I trained as a psychiatrist and the ethics remained only as a thin interest squeezed into the corners of my working life as doctor and clinical scientist. As my clinical experience grew so I became increasingly aware that ethical values lie at the heart of medicine. Much emphasis during my training was put on the importance of using scientific evidence in clinical decision-making. Little thought was given to justifying, or even noticing, the ethical assumptions that lay behind the decisions. So I moved increasingly towards medical ethics, wanting medical practice, and patients, to benefit from ethical reasoning. I enjoy the highly theoretical, and I like to pursue reasoning back towards the general and the abstract; but I keep an eye to what makes a difference in practice. I discuss the

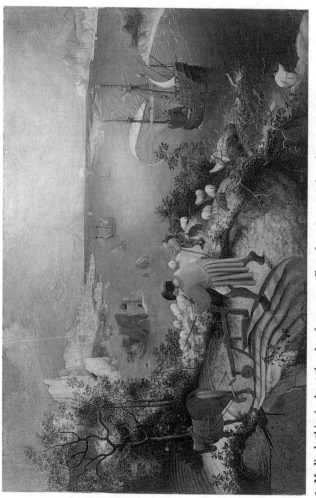

1. Medical ethics is about the ploughman as well as about Icarus (whose legs can just be seen disappearing into the sea). Bruegel, *Icarus* (1555).

philosophical minefield of the non-identity problem (Chapter 4), for example, because I believe it is relevant to decisions that doctors, and society, need to take.

The philosopher and cultural historian, Isaiah Berlin, begins an essay on Tolstoy with the following words:

> There is a line among the fragments of the Greek poet Archilocus which says: 'The fox knows many things, but the hedgehog knows one big thing'.

Berlin goes on to suggest that, taken figuratively, this distinction between the fox and the hedgehog can mark 'one of the deepest differences which divide writers and thinkers, and, it may be, human beings in general'. The hedgehog represents those who relate everything to a central vision,

> one system less or more coherent or articulate, in terms of which they understand, think and feel – a single, universal, organizing principle in terms of which alone all that they are and say has significance.

The fox represents

> those who pursue many ends, often unrelated and even contradictory, connected, if at all, only in some *de facto* way, ... [who] lead lives, perform acts, and entertain ideas that are centrifugal rather than centripetal ... seizing upon the essence of a vast variety of experiences ... without ... seeking to fit them into ... any one unchanging, all-embracing, ... unitary inner vision.

Berlin gives as examples of hedgehogs: Dante, Plato, Dostoevsky, Hegel, Proust, amongst others. He gives as examples of foxes: Shakespeare, Herodotus, Aristotle, Montaigne, and Joyce. Berlin goes on to argue that Tolstoy was a fox by nature but believed in being a hedgehog.

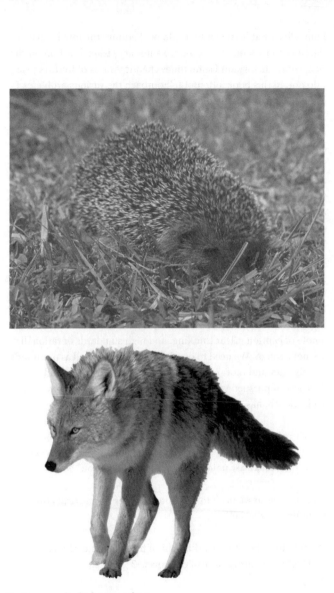

2. Are you a hedgehog or a fox?

I am a fox, or at least would like to be. I admire the intellectual rigour of those who try to produce a unitary vision, but I prefer the rich, contradictory, and sometimes chaotic visions of Berlin's foxes. I do not, in this book, attempt to approach the various problems I discuss from one single moral theory. Each chapter considers an issue on which I argue for a particular position, using whatever methods of argument seem to me to be the most relevant. I have covered different areas in different chapters: genetics, modern reproductive technologies, resource allocation, mental health, medical research, and so on; and have looked at one issue in each of these areas. At the end of the book I guide the reader to other issues and further reading. The one perspective that is common to all the chapters is the central importance of reasoning and reasonableness. I believe that medical ethics is essentially a rational subject: that is, it is all about giving reasons for the view that you take, and being prepared to change your views on the basis of reasons. That is why one chapter, in the middle of the book, is a reflection on various tools of rational argument. But although I believe in the central importance of reasons and evidence, even here the fox in me sounds a note of caution. Clear thinking, and high standards of rationality, are not enough. We need to develop our hearts as well as our minds. Consistency and moral enthusiasm can lead to bad acts and wrong decisions if pursued without the right sensitivities. The novelist, Zadie Smith, has written:

> There is no bigger crime, in the English comic novel, than thinking you are right. The lesson of the comic novel is that our moral enthusiasms make us inflexible, one-dimensional, flat.

This is a lesson we need to take into any area of practical ethics, including medical ethics.

What better place to start this tour of medical ethics than at the end, with the thorny issue of euthanasia?

Chapter 2
Euthanasia: good medical practice, or murder?

> Good deeds do not require long statements; but when evil is done
> the whole art of oratory is employed as a screen for it.
>
> (Thucydides)

The practice of euthanasia contradicts one of the oldest and most
venerated of moral injunctions: 'Thou shalt not kill'. The practice of
euthanasia, under some circumstances, is morally required by the
two most widely regarded principles that guide medical practice:
respect for patient autonomy and promoting patient's best
interests. In the Netherlands and Belgium active euthanasia
may be carried out within the law.

Outline of the requirements in order for active euthanasia to be legal in the Netherlands

1. The patient must face a future of unbearable, interminable
   suffering.
2. The request to die must be voluntary and well-considered.
3. The doctor and patient must be convinced there is no
   other solution.
4. A second medical opinion must be obtained and life must
   be ended in a medically appropriate way.

In Switzerland and in the US state of Oregon, physician-assisted suicide, that cousin of euthanasia, is legal if certain conditions are met. Three times in the last 100 years, the House of Lords in the UK has given careful consideration to the legalization of euthanasia, and on each occasion has rejected the possibility. Throughout the world, societies founded to promote voluntary euthanasia attract large numbers of members.

Playing the Nazi card

There is a common, but invalid, argument against euthanasia that I call 'playing the Nazi card'. This is when the opponent of euthanasia says to the supporter of euthanasia: 'Your views are just like those of the Nazis'. There is no need for the opponent of euthanasia to spell out the rhetorical conclusion: 'and therefore your views are totally immoral'.

Let me put the argument in a classic form used in philosophy and known as a syllogism (I will say more about syllogisms in Chapter 5):

Premise 1: Many views held by Nazis are totally immoral.
Premise 2: Your view (support for euthanasia under some
  circumstances) is one view held by Nazis.
Conclusion: Your view is totally immoral.

This is not a valid argument. It would be valid only if all the views held by Nazis were immoral.

I will therefore replace premise 1 by premise 1* as follows:

Premise 1*: All views held by Nazis are totally immoral.

In this case the argument is *logically* valid, but in order to assess whether the argument is *true* we need to assess the truth of premise 1*.

There are two possible interpretations of premise 1*. One interpretation is a version of the classic false argument known as *argumentum ad hominem* (or *bad company fallacy*): that a particular view is true or false, not because of the reasons in favour or against the view, but by virtue of the fact that a particular person (or group of people) holds that view (see Warburton, 1996). But bad people may hold some good views, and good people may hold some bad views. It is quite possible that a senior Nazi was vegetarian on moral grounds. This fact would be irrelevant to the question of whether there are, or are not, moral grounds in favour of vegetarianism. What is important are the reasons for and against the particular view, not the person who holds it. Hitler's well-known vegetarianism, by the way, was on health, not on moral, grounds (Colin Spencer, 1996).

The other, more promising, interpretation of premise 1* is that those views that are categorized as 'Nazi views' are all immoral. Some particular Nazis may hold some views about some topics that are not immoral, but those would not be 'Nazi views'. The Nazi views being referred to are a set of related views, all immoral, that are driven by racism and involve killing people against their will and against their interests. Thus, when it is said that euthanasia is a Nazi view, what is meant is that it is one of these core immoral views that characterize the immoral Nazi worldview. The problem with this argument, however, is that most supporters of euthanasia – as it is practised in the Netherlands for example – are not supporting the Nazi worldview. Quite the contrary. Those on both sides of the euthanasia debate agree that the Nazi killings that took place under the guise of 'euthanasia' were grossly immoral. The point at issue is whether euthanasia in certain specific circumstances is right or wrong, moral or immoral. All depends on being clear about these specific circumstances and being precise about what is meant by euthanasia. Only then can the arguments for and against legalizing euthanasia be properly evaluated. What is needed is some conceptual clarity.

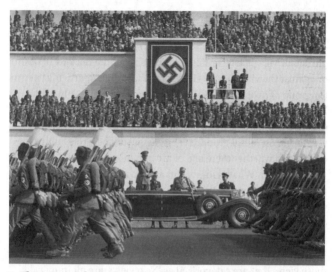

3. Those opposed to active voluntary euthanasia often play the 'Nazi card'.

Clarifying concepts in the euthanasia debate

Let us begin with some definitions (see next page). The purpose
of these is twofold: to make distinctions between different kinds
of euthanasia; and to provide us with a precise vocabulary. Such
precision is often important in evaluating arguments and reasons.
If a word is used in one sense at one point in the argument, and in
another sense at another point in the argument, then the argument
may look valid when in fact it is not.

If you study these definitions it will be immediately clear that
playing the Nazi card rides roughshod over some important
distinctions. The first point is that the term euthanasia, at least as I
am suggesting that it should be used, implies that the death is for
the person's benefit. What the Nazis did was to kill people without
any consideration of benefit to the person killed. The second point

Euthanasia and suicide: some terms

Euthanasia comes from the Greek *eu thanatos* meaning good or easy death.

Euthanasia:
X intentionally kills Y, or permits Y's death, for Y's benefit.

Active euthanasia:
X performs an action which itself results in Y's death.

Passive euthanasia:
X allows Y to die. X withholds or withdraws life-prolonging treatment.

Voluntary euthanasia:
Euthanasia when Y competently requests death himself, i.e. a competent adult wanting to die.

Non-voluntary euthanasia:
Euthanasia when Y is not competent to express a preference, e.g. Y is a severely disabled newborn.

Involuntary euthanasia:
Death is against Y's competent wishes, although X permits or imposes death for Y's benefit.

Suicide:
Y intentionally kills himself.

Assisted suicide:
X intentionally helps Y to kill himself.

Physician assisted suicide:
X (a physician) intentionally helps Y to kill himself.

> (Adapted from T. Hope, J. Savulescu, and
> J. Hendrick, *Medical Ethics and Law: The Core
> Curriculum* (Churchill Livingstone, 2003).)

is that euthanasia can be voluntary, involuntary, or non-voluntary. The third point is that it can be active or passive. Let us start with the first point.

Patients' best interests

Can it be in someone's best interests to die? I believe it can. The courts believe it can. Most doctors, nurses, and relatives believe it can. The question arises quite frequently in health care. A patient with an incurable and fatal disease may reach a stage where she will die within a day or two, but could be kept alive, with active treatment, for a few weeks more. This situation might occur because the patient gets a chest infection, or because there is a chemical imbalance in her blood, in addition to the underlying fatal disease. Antibiotics, or intravenous fluids, might treat this acute problem although they will do nothing to stop the progress of the underlying disease. All those caring for the patient will often agree that it is in the patient's best interests to die now rather than receive the life-extending treatment. The decision not to treat is even more straightforward if the patient's quality of life is now very poor, perhaps because of sustained and untreatable difficulty in breathing – a distressing feeling that is often more difficult to ameliorate than severe pain. If, however, we thought that it was in the patient's best interests to continue to live, rather than to die within days, we ought to give the life-extending treatment. But we do not think this: we believe it is in her best interests to die now rather than receive the life-extending treatment, because her quality of life, due to the underlying fatal illness, is so poor.

Respecting a patient's wishes

Most countries that put a value on individual liberty allow competent adults to refuse any medical treatment even if such treatment is in the patient's best interests; even if it is life-saving. A Jehovah's Witness, for example, may refuse a life-saving blood transfusion. If doctors were to impose treatment against the will of a competent patient then the doctor would be violating the bodily integrity of the person without consent. In legal terms this would amount to committing a 'battery'.

Passive euthanasia is widely accepted

The withholding, or withdrawing, of treatment is widely accepted as morally right in many circumstances. And it is protected in English law. There are two grounds on which it is accepted:

(1) that it is in the patient's best interests; and
(2) that it is in accord with the patient's wishes.

Either of these two conditions is sufficient reason to support passive euthanasia.

In common with widespread medical practice, I believe that there are circumstances when it is in a person's best interests to die rather than to live. I also believe that a competent person has the right to refuse life-saving treatment. Withholding or withdrawing treatment from a patient is justified in either set of circumstances, even though this will lead to death.

If I am right (and the law in England, the US, Canada, and many other countries supports this position) then why was Dr Cox, a caring English physician, convicted of attempted murder?

What Dr Cox did

Lillian Boyes was a 70-year-old patient with very severe rheumatoid arthritis. The pain seemed to be beyond the reach of painkillers. She was expected to die within a matter of days or weeks. She asked her doctor, Dr Cox, to kill her. Dr Cox injected a lethal dose of potassium chloride for two reasons:

(1) out of compassion for his patient, and

(2) because this is what she wanted him to do.

Dr Cox was charged with, and found guilty of, attempted murder. (The reason for not charging him with murder was that, given her condition, Lillian Boyes could have died from her disease and not from the injection.)

The judge, in directing the jury, said:

> Even the prosecution case acknowledged that he [Dr Cox] . . . was prompted by deep distress at Lillian Boyes' condition; by a belief that she was totally beyond recall and by an intense compassion for her fearful suffering. Nonetheless . . . if he injected her with potassium chloride for the primary purpose of killing her, or hastening her death, he is guilty of the offence charged [attempted murder] . . . neither the express wishes of the patient nor of her loving and devoted family can affect the position.

This case clearly established that active (voluntary) euthanasia is illegal (and potentially murder) under English common law. It is noteworthy that the patient was competent and wanted to be killed; close and caring relatives and her doctor (as well as the patient) believed it to be in her best interests to die, and the court did not dispute these facts.

The key difference, on which much legal and moral weight is placed, between the case of Dr Cox and the examples of withholding and withdrawing treatment that are a normal and perfectly legal part of medical practice, is that Dr Cox *killed* Lillian Boyes, and did not simply allow her to die.

Mercy killing

Moral philosophers use 'thought experiments'. These are imaginary and sometimes quite unrealistic situations that tease out and examine the morally relevant features of a situation. They are used to test the consistency of our moral beliefs. The thought experiment that I want you to consider is a case, like the Cox case, of mercy killing.

Mercy killing: the case of the trapped lorry driver

A driver is trapped in a blazing lorry. There is no way in which he can be saved. He will soon burn to death. A friend of the driver is standing by the lorry. This friend has a gun and is a good shot. The driver asks this friend to shoot him dead. It will be less painful for him to be shot than to burn to death.

I want to set aside any legal considerations and ask the purely moral question: should the friend shoot the driver?

There are two compelling reasons for the friend to kill the driver:

1. It will lead to less suffering.
2. It is what the driver wants.

These are the two reasons we have been considering with regard to justifying passive euthanasia. What reasons might you give for believing that the friend should not shoot the driver? I will consider seven reasons.

1. The friend might not kill the driver but might wound him and cause more suffering than if he had not tried to kill him.
2. There may be a chance that the driver will not burn to death but might survive the fire.
3. It is not fair on the friend in the long run: the friend will always bear the guilt of having killed the driver.
4. That although this seems to be a case where it might be right for the friend to kill the driver it would still be wrong to do so; for unless we keep strictly to the rule that killing is wrong, we will slide down a slippery slope. Soon we will be killing people when we mistakenly believe it is in their best interests. And we may slip further and kill people in our interests.

5. The argument from Nature: whereas withholding or withdrawing treatment, in the setting of a dying patient, is allowing nature to take its course, killing is an interference in Nature, and therefore wrong.

6. The argument from Playing God, which is a religious version of the argument from Nature. Killing is 'Playing God' – taking on a role that should be reserved for God alone. Letting die, on the other hand, is not usurping God's role, and may, when done with care and love, be enabling God's will to be fulfilled.

7. Killing is in principle a (great) wrong. The difference between passive euthanasia and mercy killing is that the former involves 'allowing to die' and the latter involves killing; and killing is wrong – it is a fundamental wrong.

How good are these arguments? Let's consider them one by one.

Argument 1

It is true that in real life we cannot be certain of the outcome. If you rely on argument 1 then you are not arguing that mercy killing is wrong in principle, but instead that in the real world we can never be sure that it will end in mercy. I am happy to accept that we can never be absolutely sure that the shooting will kill painlessly. There are three possible types of outcome:

(a) If the friend does not shoot (or if the bullet completely misses) then the driver will die having suffered a considerable amount of pain – let us call this amount X.

(b) The friend shoots and achieves the intended result: that the driver dies almost instantaneously and almost painlessly. In this case the driver will suffer an amount Y where Y is much smaller than X – indeed Y is almost zero if we are measuring suffering from the moment when the friend shoots.

(c) The friend shoots but only wounds the driver, causing him overall an amount of suffering Z, where Z is greater than X.

It is because of possibility (c), according to argument 1, that it would be better that the friend does not shoot the driver.

We can now compare the situation where the friend does not shoot the driver with the situation where the friend does shoot. In the former case the total amount of suffering is X. In the latter case the amount of suffering is either Y (close to zero) or Z (greater than X). Thus, by shooting, the friend may bring about a better state of affairs (less suffering) or a worse state of affairs (more suffering). If what is important is avoiding suffering, then whether it is better to shoot or not depends on the differences between X, Y, and Z and the probabilities of each of these outcomes occurring. If almost instantaneous death is by far the most likely result from shooting, and if the suffering level Z is not a great deal more than X, then it would seem right to shoot the driver because the chances are very much in favour that shooting will lead to significantly less suffering.

We can rarely be completely certain of outcomes. If this uncertainty were a reason not to act we would be completely paralysed in making decisions in life. It would be very unlikely, furthermore, that mercy killing in the medical setting (e.g. what Dr Cox did) would lead to more suffering. I conclude that argument 1 does not provide a convincing argument against voluntary active euthanasia.

Argument 2

Argument 2 is the other side of the coin from argument 1, and suffers the same weakness. The question of whether the chance that the driver might survive outweighs the greater chance that he will suffer greatly, and die, depends on what the probabilities actually are. If it is very unlikely that the driver will survive, then argument 2 is not persuasive.

Supporters of argument 2 might counter this conclusion by arguing that the weight to be given to the remote possibility of rescue from the burning lorry should be infinite. In that case, however low the probability of its occurring, the chance should be taken. There are three responses to this argument: first, what grounds are there for giving infinite weight to the possibility of rescue? Second, if we consider that very remote possibilities of rescue justify not shooting then we could equally well conclude that we should shoot. This is because it is also a remote possibility that the bullet, although intended to kill the driver, might in fact enable him to be rescued (e.g. through blowing open the cab door). Third, if argument 2 provides a convincing reason for rejecting mercy killing, it also provides a convincing reason for rejecting the withholding of medical treatment in all circumstances. This is because giving treatment might provide sufficient extension of life for a 'miracle' to occur and for the person to be cured and live healthily for very much longer.

Argument 3

The third argument fails because it begs the very question that is under debate. The friend should only feel guilt if shooting the driver were the wrong thing to do. But the point at issue is what is the right and wrong thing to do. If it is right to shoot the driver, then the friend should not feel guilty if he shot him (thus reducing the driver's suffering). The possibility of guilt is not a reason, one way or the other, for deciding how the friend should act. Rather we first have to answer the question of what is the right thing to do and only then can we ask whether the friend ought to feel guilty.

Argument 4

Argument 4 is a version of what is known as the 'slippery slope argument'. This is such an important type of argument in medical ethics that I will consider it in more detail in Chapter 5. I will distinguish two types of slippery slope – the logical, or conceptual, slope; and the empirical, or in-practice, slope. The types of reason needed to counter a slippery slope argument depend, as we shall see, on which type of argument is being advanced.

Arguments 5 and 6

The arguments from Nature and from Playing God have, like the slippery slope argument, a more general application in medical ethics. I will consider them in more detail later (Chapter 5).

Argument 7

Of all the arguments considered, it is only argument 7 that views killing as wrong in principle.

Is mercy killing wrong in principle?

At this stage we need to get clear what 'killing' means. Those who believe that mercy killing, but not the common medical practice of passive euthanasia, is wrong in principle do so on the grounds that mercy killing involves *actively* causing death rather than failing to prevent it.

But this is not sufficient. Consider the following medical situation. Morphine is sometimes given to patients close to death from an untreatable illness, in order to ensure that the patient suffers as little pain as possible. In addition to preventing pain, morphine also reduces the depth and frequency of breathing (through its action on the part of the brain that controls respiration). In some situations, although not all, morphine can have the foreseeable effect of shortening the patient's life, as well as reducing pain. A doctor who gave morphine to a terminally ill patient in order to reduce the suffering of the patient and foreseeing (although not intending) the earlier death of the patient, would not have broken the law. Indeed, giving morphine in these circumstances is often good clinical practice. And yet injecting morphine into a patient is just as active a thing to do as is injecting potassium chloride. The key difference is that, in the case of potassium chloride, the *intention* is for the patient to die – and this is the means to reducing the patient's suffering. In the case of morphine the intention is to relieve the pain; an earlier death is *foreseen but not intended*. That is,

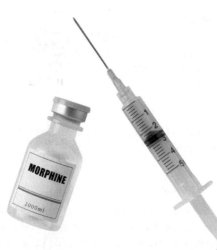

4. Dr A injects morphine (a powerful painkiller) intending to relieve pain and suffering for a dying patient, and foreseeing that the patient may die more quickly. Dr B injects morphine to hasten a dying patient's death in order to relieve pain and suffering. Is there a moral difference between what Dr A does and what Dr B does?

at any rate, how the law in England and many other countries sees it.

On this analysis, killing, as in mercy killing, involves two aspects: that what is done is a positive act (rather than simply an omission to act); and that death is intended (and not simply foreseen). Both these aspects are necessary to the definition of killing but neither by itself is sufficient.

In short, the argument to the effect that mercy killing is wrong in principle puts great moral importance on (1) the distinction between acts and omissions; and (2) the distinction between intending and foreseeing the death. Both the question of whether there is a moral, or even a conceptual, difference between acts and omissions on the one hand, or between intention and foresight on

Hypothetical cases (thought experiments) to examine the moral importance of the distinction between acts and omissions; and between intending and foreseeing an outcome

1. The cases of Smith and Jones
Smith sneaks into the bathroom of his 6-year-old cousin and drowns him, arranging things so that it will look like an accident. The reason Smith does this is that the death of his cousin will result in his coming into a large inheritance.

Jones stands to gain a similar large inheritance from the death of his 6-year-old cousin. Like Smith, Jones sneaks into the bathroom with the intention of drowning his cousin. The cousin, however, accidentally slips and knocks his head and drowns in the bath. Jones could easily have saved his cousin, but far from trying to save him, he stands ready to push the child's head back under. However, this does not prove necessary.

Is there a moral difference between Smith's and Jones's behaviour?

This pair of cases is used to support the view that there is no moral distinction between an act (killing) and an omission (failing to save) when the outcome and intention are the same.

2. The cases of Robinson and Davies
Robinson does not give £100 to a charity that is helping to combat starvation in a poor country. As a result, one person dies of starvation who would have lived had Robinson sent the money.

Davies does send £100 but also sends a poisoned food parcel for use by a charity that distributes food donations. The overall and intended result is that one person is killed from the poisoned food parcel and another person's life is saved by the £100 donation.

Is there a moral difference between what Robinson and Davies do? If there is, is this because Davies acts to kill, whereas Robinson only omits to act?

This pair of cases is used to counter the conclusion from the cases of Smith and Jones and to show that, even when the overall outcome is the same, an act (sending the poison parcel) together with the intention to kill is morally very much worse than the omission (failing to send charitable aid).

3. Sacrificing one to save five

The runaway train: A runaway train is approaching points on the railway line. If the points are not switched then the train will kill five people who are strapped to the line. If the points are switched the train will go along a different line and kill just one (different) person. There is no way of stopping the train; but you can switch the points so that one person, rather than five people, dies.

Should you switch the points?

Organ donation: One healthy person could be killed in order to use his organs to save the lives of five people with various types of organ failure.

Should you kill the healthy person and use his organs?

A common intuition is that it would be right to switch the points in the first case (so that fewer people die) but wrong to kill the healthy person in order to use his organs to save more lives. In both cases, however, by not acting five people die and by acting only one person dies. What justifies the common intuitions? This pair of examples is used in support of the view that the nature of the act can make enormous moral difference even when the outcome is the same.

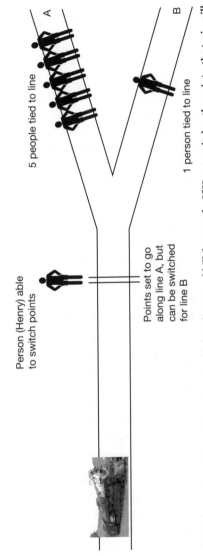

A

5 people tied to line

Person (Henry) able
to switch points

Points set to go
along line A, but
can be switched
for line B

B

1 person tied to line

5. If Henry does nothing, the train will run along line A and kill five people. If Henry switches the points, the train will run along line B and kill one (different) person. The train cannot be stopped in time, nor can any of the six people tied to a rail track be released in time. Should Henry switch the points?

the other, have been much debated, and no single definitive position is generally agreed. The preceding box gives some of the thought experiments used by both sides in the argument. I do not want to discuss the general question of these moral distinctions – only where they are relevant to the euthanasia debate.

It is noteworthy that all these thought experiments involve killing, or failing to save, that is not for a person's benefit. Some of the examples, furthermore, involve killing one person to save another. In the setting of euthanasia, of course, this is not the situation. I know of no convincing thought experiment that shows a moral distinction between acts and omissions, or intention and foresight, which includes the following three key features of euthanasia:

(1) that the person whose act we are evaluating has a clear duty of care to the person who dies;
(2) that there is no issue of harming one person to benefit another;
(3) where death is in the best interests of the person who dies.

It is the harm of death that makes killing wrong

Opponents of euthanasia may ultimately rest their case on one basic principle: killing is morally wrong. They may accept that there are difficult cases when killing one person may save another – or many others. They may accept that in such circumstances killing may be the right thing to do. But in the case of euthanasia, no other person's life will be saved. The wrong of euthanasia is based on the wrong of killing, and is not balanced by saving any other life.

It is right that we have a strong intuition that killing is wrong. For most people dying now would be a great harm compared with continuing to live. The reason why killing is normally a great wrong is that dying is normally a great harm. The wrong of killing, however, is a result of the harm of dying, not vice versa. If, therefore, it is in the best interests of a patient to die now rather than suffer a prolonged and painful dying, then killing is no longer a wrong. In other words when death is a benefit, and not a harm, then killing is not a wrong. Those who argue that mercy killing is wrong in principle forget the conceptual link between the wrong of killing and harm of dying.

Conclusion

I reject the view that voluntary active euthanasia is wrong in principle on the grounds that this argument puts the cart before the horse: it is the harm of dying that makes killing a wrong and not the other way round. When suffering is the result of following a moral principle then we need to look very carefully at our moral principle and ask whether we are applying it too inflexibly. I believe this is what we are doing when we claim that voluntary active euthanasia is morally wrong. It is perverse to seek a sense of moral purity when this is gained at the expense of the suffering of others.

Euthanasia

Chapter 3
Why undervaluing 'statistical' people costs lives

Whether happiness be or be not the end to which morality should be referred – that it should be referred to an end of some sort, and not left in the dominion of vague feeling or inexplicable internal conviction, that it be made a matter of reason and calculation, and not merely of sentiment, is essential to the very idea of moral philosophy . . .

(J. S. Mill, *London and Westminster Review*, 1838)

The cash value of life

In January 1997 Tony Bullimore was attempting to sail round the world in the Vendée Globe race. He had reached the dangerous and cold waters of the Southern Ocean, over 1,500 miles south of the Australian coast, when his boat was capsized by hurricane force winds and enormous waves. He spent four days trapped under its hull before he was rescued in the largest and most expensive such operation ever undertaken by the Australian defence forces. How much money should a civilized society be prepared to spend in order to save a life? Is the answer 'whatever it takes', or should there be a limit? When is the chance of success too low even to attempt a costly rescue operation?

Let me pose a more general question. What is the cash value of a human life? This question is a disturbing one to ask but,

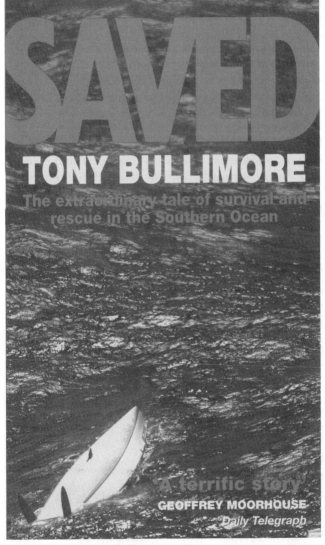

SAVED

TONY BULLIMORE

The extraordinary tale of survival and
rescue in the Southern Ocean

'A terrific story'
GEOFFREY MOORHOUSE
Daily Telegraph

6. How much money should a civilized society be prepared to spend in
order to save the life of one person?

paradoxically, there are situations where avoiding the question may cost lives, and allocating scarce medical resources is one of them.

There is no health care system in the world that has sufficient money to provide the best possible treatment for all patients in all situations, not even those that spend relatively large sums on health care (see box). New and better treatments are being developed all the time. On average, in the UK, about three new medicines are licensed each month. Almost all have some benefit over existing treatments and some will extend people's lives. Many of these new medicines are expensive. When is the extra benefit worth the extra cost? This question must be asked by all health care systems, whether private systems, such as 'managed care' in the US, or publicly funded systems, such as the British National Health Service.

If the best treatment cannot always be provided then choices have to be made. The general question of how our limited health care resources should be distributed is one of the most important in

National expenditure on health: examples of some of the wealthier nations

Country	% GDP	per capita purchasing power ($)
Australia	8.6	2085
Canada	9.3	2360
France	9.4	2043
Germany	10.3	2361
New Zealand	8.1	1440
Norway	9.4	2452
United Kingdom	6.8	1510
United States	12.9	4165

Data, for 1998, from OECD Health Data 2001

medical ethics. The quality and quantity of thousands of people's lives will be affected by the answers that we give.

Quality of life

Some medical treatments have little or no effect on life-span but improve quality of life: hip replacement for osteoarthritis is an example. One rather deep problem that faces us in thinking about the right way to distribute health resources is how we compare and evaluate the relative importance of improving quality of life *vis-à-vis* extending it. I am not going to tackle this issue, nor the problems associated with the measurements of quality of life in the first place. I will focus exclusively on life-extending treatments since there are more than enough problems in thinking about allocating resources to these treatments alone. There are many examples of life-extending treatments. Surgery for appendicitis extends life because without such surgery most people would die. Breast cancer screening can extend life because early detection and treatment can increase life-span. High blood pressure increases the risk of death from heart attack and stroke. Treatment that lowers blood pressure reduces, although it does not eliminate, this risk. Renal dialysis keeps those people alive whose kidneys no longer function adequately. Each year of dialysis is a year more life.

In control of a budget

Imagine that you are in charge of a health service for a particular population. You have a limited budget – you cannot afford the best treatment for all of the people all of the time. You have decided how to spend most of your budget and you have a few hundred thousand pounds left uncommitted. You sit down with your advisers to consider the best way of spending this last remaining tranche of money. There are three possibilities and you must choose one of them. The possibilities are:

(1) a new treatment for bowel cancer that gives the relevant patients a small but significant chance of increased life-expectancy;

(2) a new drug that lowers the chance of death from heart attack in people with genetically induced raised blood cholesterol;

(3) a new piece of surgical kit that ensures a lower mortality from a particularly difficult kind of brain surgery.

On what basis do you choose between these possibilities?

One approach that has a lot going for it is to say: there is no good reason to prefer one person's year of life over another person's, or to give any priority to people who would benefit from the bowel cancer treatment over people who have the genetically induced high blood cholesterol or to people with the brain tumour. In each case people stand to die prematurely and in each case the treatment increases the chance that they will live for longer. What we should do, therefore, is to spend the money so that we can 'buy' as many life years as possible. By doing this we are treating everyone fairly: we are valuing one year of life equally, regardless of whose life it is.

The distribution problem

Even amongst people (like me) who are attracted by this approach there is an issue that needs to be faced: the 'distribution problem'. Take a look at the three interventions described in the box.

Choosing between three interventions		
Intervention 1	**benefits 10 people**	total life years gained: 35
Intervention 2	**benefits 15 people**	total life years gained: 30
Intervention 3	**benefits 2 people**	total life years gained: 16

Suppose that all these interventions cost the same and that we can only afford one of them. Suppose further that the distributions are as follows. The two people who are benefited by intervention 3 will enjoy 8 more years of life each. Of the ten people who are benefited by intervention 1, the average benefit is 3.5 years and the range is 2–4 years. Of the fifteen people who are benefited by intervention 2, the average benefit is 2 years and the range is 1 to 3 years. Which of the three interventions should we go for?

If we think that what we should do is to 'buy' the maximum number of life years that we can (the maximization view) then we should put our money into intervention 1 because we buy 35 life years, which is more than we will get if we spend the money on either of the other two interventions. Some might argue that intervention 2 is preferable because we help more people (15 as opposed to 10) although each person gains fewer extra years of life. Still others might argue that intervention 3 is the best option because the two people who are helped receive a really significant gain (eight years of life) whereas no one gains more than four years of life with either of the other two options. The question of whether it is only the total number of life years that matters, or whether the way in which those years are distributed between people is important, is known as 'the distribution problem'. Those who reject the maximization view have to specify how they balance the value in helping more people, but each gaining relatively less, against the value in helping fewer people, but each gaining relatively more. Except at extremes I am generally happy to go with maximizing the total number of life years and not worry too much about their distribution.

In being generally happy with using resources to maximize total number of life years I am in a minority – and no health care system in the world behaves remotely in this way. One problem with my position (the maximization view) takes us right back to Tony Bullimore and his attempt to sail round the world. My position gives no moral weight to what has been called 'The Rule of Rescue' – and yet this rule seems, intuitively, to be right.

The rule of rescue

The 'rule of rescue' is relevant to a situation where there is an identified person whose life is at high risk. There exists an intervention ('rescue') which has a good chance of saving the person's life. The value that is at the heart of 'the rule of rescue' is this: that it is normally justified to spend more per life year gained in this situation than in situations where we cannot identify who has been helped.

Consider two hypothetical, but realistic, situations in health care.

Intervention A (saves anonymous 'statistical' lives)

A is a drug which will change the chance of death by a small amount in a large number of people. For example, out of every 2,000 people in the relevant group, if A is not given then 100 people will die over the next few years. If A is given then only 98 will die. Although we know that drug A will prevent deaths we do not know which specific lives will be saved. Drug A is cheap – the cost per life year gained is £20,000. One example of a medical treatment like this is treatment that lowers moderately raised blood pressure. Another example is a class of medicines known as statins that lower blood cholesterol. Lowering blood pressure, and lowering cholesterol, reduce risk of heart attack, stroke, and death.

Intervention B (rescues an identified person)

B is the only effective treatment for an otherwise life-threatening condition. Those with the condition face a greater than 90 per cent chance of death over the next year if not given B. If given B then there is a good chance of cure – say 90 per cent. B is expensive. The cost per life year gained is £50,000. Renal (kidney) dialysis is an example of this type.

There are three, potentially relevant, differences between intervention A and intervention B. The first is that B saves lives within the next year, whereas the benefits of A are not realized for many years. This difference has some moral relevance. A few of those who might benefit from intervention A will die from some quite independent cause before any benefit from A could be gained. There are also problems in calculating the cost per life year gained when at least some of the costs of the intervention are borne years before the benefits are seen. This is because of monetary inflation. Both these effects can be allowed for in the calculation of cost per life year gained. Having made such allowances, there seems no good reason to value the saving of life years in the future any less than saving life years now.

The second difference between the interventions is that B will almost certainly save the lives of the relevant patients, but A only has a low probability of doing so. Thus B might be seen as giving greater benefit to individuals than A. I will argue, in a moment, that this is false.

The third difference is that intervention B benefits identifiable people. Intervention A benefits a proportion of patients within a group (e.g. those with raised blood pressure), but we cannot know who within the group will benefit (although we may know the likely proportion that will benefit).

According to the rule of rescue it may be right for a health care system to fund intervention B but not intervention A, even though B is more expensive in terms of life years gained. For example, the rule of rescue would provide justification for spending more per life year gained on treatments such as renal replacement therapy, than on treatments like statins.

In practice this is exactly what health care systems do. The British National Health Service provides renal dialysis at costs over £50,000 per life year gained, whilst paying for statins only for those with very high cholesterol levels. This is despite the fact that treatment with statins for those with moderately raised cholesterol levels would cost only about £10,000 per life year gained. In other words, if the money spent on some people for renal dialysis were, instead, spent on some people with moderately raised cholesterol, five times as many life years could be gained. But we don't do it – because we would feel that we had condemned the person needing dialysis to death; whereas all we would be doing in the case of statins is slightly lowering an already quite small chance of death.

The most powerful reason in support of the rule of rescue is that in the typical case the identified person, like Tony Bullimore, stands to gain a significant increase in chance of life, whereas in the typical case of saving anonymous 'statistical' lives no one stands to gain more than a small decrease in probability of death. I will put this argument in favour of the rule of rescue as strongly as I can. I will then say why I do not agree with it.

The strongest argument in favour of the rule of rescue

Premature death is, normally, a very significant harm indeed. But a very small chance of premature death is by no means a great harm – and we cannot claim that we need something which reduces by a very small amount the chance of premature death. All of us in our lives trade small increases in the chance of premature death against really quite small benefits. Consider the Sunday morning cyclist.

The Sunday morning cyclist

On Sunday mornings I cycle along the busy Banbury Road in my home town of Oxford to buy a newspaper. In doing this I am putting myself at (what I hope is) only a small extra risk of premature death. I am trading this extra risk against the pleasure and value of reading the Sunday morning paper. In balancing these two I find that the pleasure of the paper – a really rather small pleasure in my life – outweighs the extra risk of premature death. There seems nothing irrational in this. A very small chance of a terrible harm is itself only a small negative weight easily outweighed by other benefits.

34

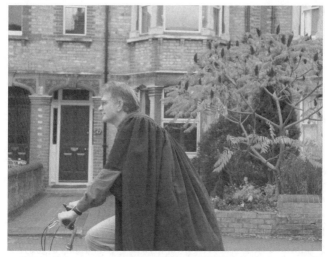

7. **The Sunday morning cyclist on the way to buy a newspaper: a small extra risk of death is offset by the pleasure of reading the paper.**

Most of us will take these small risks not only for our own benefit but for the benefit of others. Consider the friend's job application.

The friend's job application

Suppose that a friend is applying for a job which he is keen to get. To meet the application deadline it has to be in the postbox today. Owing to a severe bout of influenza, my friend cannot post it himself. To help him I cycle to his house to collect the application and post it. Again, this action increases by a very small amount my chance of premature death. This is easily outweighed by the value of helping my friend.

With these considerations in mind I will propose an argument in favour of a health care system paying for a 'rescue' intervention of type B (at, for example, a cost of £50,000 per life year gained) whilst refusing to pay for an anonymous 'statistical' intervention of type A (at, for example, a cost of only £20,000 per life year gained).

I will make the argument using the cholesterol-lowering drugs (statins) as an example of the anonymous 'statistical' intervention, and renal dialysis as an example of the rescue intervention.

Those who would benefit from treatment with statins gain very little – a very small reduction in the risk of premature death. The 'friend's job application' shows that we readily risk small changes in the chance of premature death, even for benefits to other people. If we ourselves stood to gain from the statins treatment (because we had moderately raised cholesterol levels) it would be reasonable, and not extraordinarily altruistic, for us to prefer that the money go not to provide us with statins but towards the cost of renal dialysis for someone who would otherwise die. From the point of view of those who have to decide how limited health care resources should be distributed, it certainly seems better to keep a few people alive (who would otherwise certainly die) than to reduce only slightly the chance of death of a large number of people, particularly when the risk of premature death is fairly low anyway.

Back to the distribution problem

The rule of rescue seems to be a particular example of the distribution problem. Most people reject maximizing life years gained (which would favour paying for statin treatment). Essentially, the intuitive appeal is as follows: it is better to provide a great benefit (continuing life in people who would otherwise certainly die) to a few people than a trivial benefit (a small reduction in chance of premature death) in a large number of people.

Why I disagree with the rule of rescue

Despite the strong intuitive appeal of the rule of rescue, and the arguments that I have outlined in favour of it, I stick by my preference for maximizing benefit. I will argue for my position by considering a counter-example to this conclusion: the case of the trapped miner.

The case of the trapped miner

Consider the case of the trapped miner (see box). Suppose that the facts are these (perhaps not entirely realistic). There is a small risk of death to those in the rescue party, and this risk varies according to the size of the rescue party. If there were 100 rescuers there would be a 1:1,000 chance for each rescuer of death. If there were 1,000 rescuers each would face a 1:2,000 chance of death. If 10,000 rescuers then each would face a 1:5,000 chance of death. If 100,000 rescuers (an extraordinarily large rescue party – but this is a 'thought experiment' to test a theoretical point) then each would face a 1:10,000 risk.

Thus, the larger the size of the rescue party, the smaller the risk of death faced by each individual rescuer. It is also the case, however, that the larger the size of the rescue party, the more people are likely to die in the rescue attempt. With a rescue party of 100,000, each member of the rescue party faces a very small risk of death – well within the risks that we normally take for much less important gains than saving a life. However, with such a rescue party, about ten people are likely to die in order to save the life of the one trapped miner.

The case of the trapped miner

A miner lies trapped following an accident. Without rescue he will die. Given a sufficiently large rescue party the miner can be saved.

Take a moment to consider the following questions:

1. Do you think you should join the rescue party if you faced a 1:10,000 risk of death in so doing?
2. Is there any further key information you need to know before you can answer the first question?

If we assume that most people are altruistic at least to a small extent, and most people will accept a very small level of risk of personal death in order to save another's life; and if we assume, further, that most people, given the choice, would like to face as low a personal risk of death as possible, then respecting the wishes of each potential member of the rescue party would have the following result. The wishes of potential members of the rescue party would be most respected by putting together an enormous rescue party in order to save the trapped miner – at the expense of many lives.

Thus, if the issue of rescue is seen simply as a question of balancing individual risks for each rescuer against the benefit to the individual of being rescued, then it would seem right to pursue a policy which overall was very costly in terms of lives lost.

Suppose that a senior army officer will lead the rescue. If that army officer were to coordinate the rescue, with the foreseeable result that more people would die in the attempt to rescue than would be saved by the rescue, then the army officer might reasonably be criticized, even if the rescue party were made up entirely of

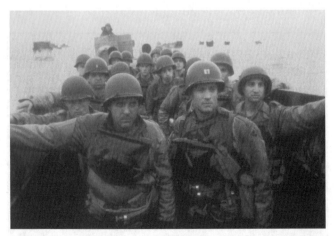

8. **Saving Private Ryan: should the lives of many be risked to save one?**

volunteers who knew and accepted the risk to themselves. He would have been responsible for a rescue operation that caused, and had been expected to cause, more deaths amongst the rescuers than the number of people who were rescued. Leading such a rescue even with fully informed volunteers is highly problematic from a moral point of view.

Further key information

Let me return to the second question I asked about the case of the trapped miner: is there any further key information you need before answering the first question? I think you should know not only your personal risk in joining the rescue party, but also the size of the rescue party. Because if the rescue party needs only ten people and each member has a risk of 1:10,000 of dying then the miner's life will be saved with (almost certainly) no loss of life. But if the rescue party needs to be 100,000 strong then almost certainly many lives will be lost in rescuing the one miner. I would be much happier (from the moral point of view) volunteering for the first rescue party than the second.

Back to health care

Let us reconsider statins and renal dialysis. It is not clear that those who could benefit from the anonymous 'statistical' intervention (e.g. statins) have voluntarily agreed to forgo their treatment in order for identifiable patients to receive expensive life-extending treatment. A health care system that spends more per year of life gained on rescue treatments (such as renal dialysis) than on 'statistical' treatments is effectively volunteering those who would benefit from the preventive treatment to take part in a 'rescue party' for those requiring the rescue treatment. Because of limited resources, any health care system, in making decisions about treatments which extend people's lives, has to extend some people's lives at the expense of other people's lives. In the absence of a clear mandate from the group of people who stand to lose by a particular decision, it seems to me that the core principle must be that those decisions should be taken which overall maximize the number of life years gained. And even if there were such a clear mandate (which there is not) it remains questionable, as with the army officer leading the rescue operation with fully informed volunteers, whether it would be right for a health care system to let more die to save fewer.

A counter-intuitive conclusion

But can we accept this conclusion? Let's go back to Tony Bullimore and the dramatic and successful rescue undertaken by the Australian defence forces. Only a stone-hearted theorist could read Bullimore's account and conclude that it was wrong to mount such a rescue. The Australian defence forces were right to spend millions of tax-payers' dollars. In the same way it is right for a society to spend £50,000 a year to keep a patient alive on renal dialysis. How could we stand by and say to a patient: we could keep you alive for many years but we will not provide the necessary money – we have other priorities. And how could we say this to the relatives who would be bereaved?

This seems very different from the situation of the patient with moderately raised cholesterol. Without treatment the chances are that the person will not have a heart attack and die. By refusing the treatment we are not condemning him to death as we are the person who needs renal dialysis.

But the logic of the case of the trapped miner refutes this. It is true that if we do not provide treatment for the raised cholesterol we will not know which specific people die as a result of lack of treatment, nor which relatives have been bereaved. But we do know that there are such people.

Enlarging our moral imagination

So how do we square the circle? What do we learn from our empathy with Tony Bullimore or a person with renal failure? The answer, I think, is not that we should become stone-hearted logicians and refuse to attempt the rescue of Bullimore or to provide renal dialysis. It is right that our moral imagination and our human sympathy are awakened. What we should learn from the logic of the case of the trapped miner is that our moral imagination must also be awake to the sadness of lives cut short, and relatives bereaved, because we did not provide treatment for moderately raised cholesterol. Deaths are not less significant because we cannot put a face or a name to the person whose life could have been saved.

Health care is good value for money. The lesson we should learn from our empathy for those in need of rescue is to widen our moral imaginations. We rightly respond to the person in distress by being prepared to spend money to save a life. We should respond in the same way to prevent 'statistical' deaths, for such deaths are real people and the friends and relatives who are left behind mourn in just the same way.

Chapter 4
People who don't exist; at least not yet

> The minutest philosophers, who, by the by, have the most enlarged understandings, (their souls being inversely as their enquiries) shew us incontestably, the HOMUNCULUS ... may be benefited, – he may be injured, – he may obtain redress; – in a word, he has all the claims and rights of humanity, which *Tully*, *Puffendorf*, or the best ethick writers allow to arise out of that state and relation.

The story of medical ethics begins before conception. In the opinion of Tristram Shandy, a person's character, and the life he will enjoy, is shaped by the parents' thoughts during copulation. Tristram complains:

> I wish either my father or my mother, or indeed both of them, as they were in duty both equally bound to it, had minded what they were about when they begot me; had they duly consider'd how much depended upon what they were then doing; – that not only the production of a rational Being was concerned in it; but that possibly the happy formation and temperature of his body, perhaps his genius and the very cast of his mind: – and, for aught they knew to the contrary, even the fortunes of his whole house might take their turn from the humours and dispositions which were then uppermost ... *Pray, my Dear*, quoth my mother, *have you not forgot to wind up the clock? – Good G—!* cried my father, making an exclamation, but taking care to moderate his voice at the same time,

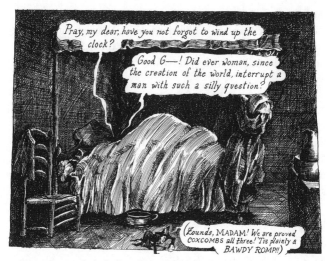

9. Doctors must 'mind what they are about' when they help a woman to conceive.

– Did ever woman, since the creation of the world, interrupt a man with such a silly question?

The Human Fertilisation and Embryology Act 1990 (HFEA) – the law that governs assisted reproduction services in the UK – requires doctors to mind what they are about when they help a woman to conceive a child. The Act states: 'A woman shall not be provided with treatment services unless account has been taken of the welfare of any child who may be born as a result of the treatment (including the need of that child for a father) . . . '

A great deal of brouhaha was created in the British press when a post-menopausal woman aged 59 years went to a private fertility clinic in Italy to be helped to conceive a child (in fact she subsequently gave birth to twins). 'Think of the poor children who will be born' was one response 'they will be the laughing stock of their friends when they are met at

43

the school gate by such an elderly mother'. According to one member of the Human Fertilisation and Embryology Authority (which oversees fertility clinics), concern for the welfare of the potential children rules out fertility treatment for elderly women.

The welfare of children is so important a consideration in our moral thinking that the wording of the HFEA may seem unproblematic: but this is not so. When assisting conception it is not the welfare of an actual child that is under consideration, it is the welfare of a child that may exist at a later time, if indeed there will later exist any such child at all. It turns out that a consideration of the welfare of children who may exist at a later time is a very slippery customer indeed.

The analogy with adoption

In the early days of in-vitro fertilization (IVF) – the technique that led to the idea of test-tube babies – a Manchester woman was removed from the IVF waiting list when it was discovered that she had a criminal record involving prostitution offences. The hospital concerned had a policy in place (this was a couple of years before the HFEA was enacted). This policy stated that couples wanting IVF 'must in the ordinary course of events, satisfy the general criteria established by adoption societies in assessing suitability for adoption'.

In effect this policy means that if a person seeking IVF would not be considered suitable as an adoptive parent, she should not be provided with assistance to reproduce. And underlying this policy, presumably, is the idea of the welfare of the child who might exist at a later time. But does the analogy between adoption and assisting reproduction hold?

In the case of adoption we have a child (child X) and a number of possible adoptive parents: A, B, C etc. Suppose that we have good

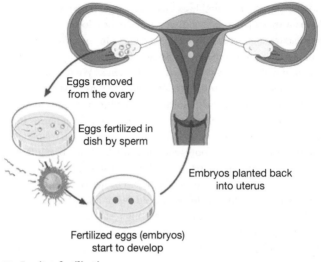

Eggs removed
from the ovary

Eggs fertilized in
dish by sperm

Embryos planted back
into uterus

Fertilized eggs (embryos)
start to develop

10. In-vitro fertilization.

reason to believe that parents A will be better parents than B, C, etc. and that child X is likely to have a better life if we choose parents A than if we choose any of the other parents (B, C, etc.). Assuming that judgements about the likely quality of parenting can be made (and such judgements have to be made by adoption agencies) then we act, as far as we can judge, in child X's best interests in giving child X to parents A.

Now compare this situation of adoption with that of assisting reproduction. Suppose that couples A, B, C, etc. come for help with fertility treatment. All these couples are likely to be perfectly reasonable parents but we have good reason to believe that couple A are likely to be better parents than couples B, C, etc. Which couple should we help? Would we not be acting in the best interests of the child who may come to exist if we helped parents A, on the grounds that, as far as we can judge, the child would be happier with couple A than with couples B, C, etc.?

It is not, however, as simple as this. There is no kingdom, as far as I am aware, of potential children waiting to be allocated to a particular set of parents. If we help couple A to conceive, then one child (child a) will come into existence. If we help couple B then a different child (child b) will come into existence. What sense can we make of assessing the interests of the child that may exist at a later time? If we help couple B then child b would come to exist and have a good start in life but not as good as child a would have done. If we have the resources to help only one couple, which couple should we choose, if our only criterion is what is in the best interests of the child who will come to exist? It is tempting to say that the best interests of the child would be served by helping couple A. But this is wrong. It will be a different child depending on which couple we help. It is in potential child a's best interests for us to help couple A, but in potential child b's best interests to help couple B. If we focus on the interests of the child who may exist at a later date the question that needs to be asked is: are these interests better served if he or she is born to these parents or if he or she never exists at all? The question, put this way, is of course rather odd since it asks us to compare existence with non-existence. Perhaps a better question is: if there were later to exist a child to this couple, would it have a reasonable expectation of a life worth living? I will come back to these issues in the next section. The key point for the present discussion is that the possibility of 'this' potential child being born to any other (possibly better) parents does not arise. This, crucially, is where the analogy with adoption breaks down.

If we have the resources to help only one couple then an argument could be made for choosing to help couple A. The argument is as follows: if we help couple A then the child that will exist (child a) will be happier (on the best prediction) than the child (child b) who would have existed had we helped couple B. If there are no other relevant grounds for choosing between the various couples then it is better to act in such a way as to bring about the existence of the happiest children that we can. We are, in this case, most likely to bring about the existence of the happiest child that we can by helping couple A rather than couples B, C, etc. We should, therefore, help couple A. In choosing to help couple A we are acting *against* the best interests of the child who would have existed in the future had we helped couple B instead. Our choice to help couple A is not on the grounds of an individual's best interests but in order to make the world a better place. The child who will actually exist in that 'better world' (i.e. child *a*) will have a better life than the different child (child *b*) who would have existed had we helped couple B rather than couple A.

This point can be made more strongly by considering the following analogy. Suppose that a hospital delays the admission of a patient who requires non-urgent surgery in order to admit a patient

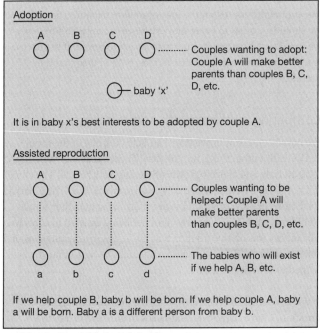

11. **Adoption vs assisted reproduction.**

requiring an urgent operation. No one would maintain that it was in the best interests of the first patient that her surgery be delayed. On the contrary, it is against her best interests. The justification for acting against her best interests is in order to benefit the patient who needs urgent surgery. Since a choice has to be made, the decision to give priority to the patient in more urgent need seems the right one.

We seem to have found an argument that justifies the initial intuition that, in the case of assisting reproduction, we should help couple A rather than couples B, C, etc. (assuming that we have the resources to help one only). This argument is not based on the idea of acting in the best interests of the child who may be born. It is not based on following the guidelines from the HFEA or from St Mary's Hospital in Manchester. Instead, the argument is based on the idea of welfare maximization: that we should act so as to bring into existence as happy children as we can. Does it matter that the reasons are different, if the decision is the same? The answer is that it does, both in theory and in practice.

Comparing existence with non-existence

We have been assuming that we can help only one of the couples A, B, C, etc. But often this is not the case. The 59-year-old woman who went to Italy and conceived twins bore the costs herself. The clinic did not have to choose between her and someone else. The outcry in the British press was not on the grounds that some other couple would not receive help as a result of her being assisted to conceive. The outcry was on the grounds that it was against the interests of the potential child (i.e. any child who might be born) that she be helped to conceive at all.

If we focus solely on the interests of the potential child, the question, I have suggested, that needs to be asked is: are the interests of this potential child better served if he or she is born to

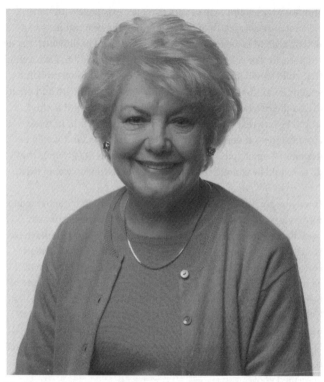

12. Should a 59-year-old post-menopausal woman be helped to have a child using assisted reproduction?

these parents, or if he or she never exists at all? But this is a very strange question. Does it make any sense to compare existence (in whatever state) with non-existence? Some have said such a comparison is like dividing by zero – it appears to make sense at first sight, but it is a function without meaning. Others think that as long as the child will not have an appalling life then it is in the child's best interests to exist, on the grounds that, on the whole, existence is a positive thing. Perhaps some, like Montesquieu, of a more pessimistic disposition, take the opposite view and see existence, on balance, as a negative experience.

If those who say that one cannot compare existence with non-existence are correct, then the criterion of the best interests of a potential child is meaningless. But this view faces a difficulty. Let us suppose, for the sake of argument, that were couple J to have a child that child would suffer immensely (perhaps from some dreadful genetic condition). The child would live in constant pain and finally die, to the relief of all, at the age of one. So the life of this child would be one year of constant pain followed by death. In these circumstances it does seem to make sense to say that it would be wrong to help couple J conceive such a child on the grounds that to do so would be against the interests of the child who would exist.

It may be possible to make sense of this judgement without having to 'divide by zero'. Over any period of life one can ask whether, overall, the experiences are positive or negative. The zero line here is such that life above zero is overall worth living for the person concerned and life below zero is not worth living. In the case of the child who would be born to couple J, his life, overall, would rate as below zero. It is for this reason that we can say that it is in his best interests not to be born. In saying this we do not rely on the problematic comparison of non-existence with existence, but on being able to make a judgement as to whether the life it is predicted that he would have would, overall, be above or below zero (as described above).

The argument that the post-menopausal 59-year-old woman should not be helped to conceive, on the grounds that to do so would be against the best interests of the potential child, falls apart, whichever view you take on this issue.

1. If it makes no sense to compare existence with non-existence then it makes no sense to argue that in helping the woman conceive one is acting against the best interests of the potential child. For on this view one cannot argue anything on the basis of best interests, since on this view it is meaningless to compare the interests in not existing with the interests in existing.

2. If, on the other hand, it does make sense to judge whether it is in the interests of a child (who may exist in the future) to exist, and if that judgement is essentially whether the predicted life will be, overall, a positive experience, then the question to be asked is this: is the predicted life of a child born to this 59-year-old woman, overall, likely to be positive?

If, like me on a bad day, you take a rather gloomy view of existence, then perhaps you think it is not in the interests of the child, who may come to exist, for the woman to be helped to conceive. But it was not such a view that prompted the outcry against helping the post-menopausal woman to conceive. Such a view would, after all, justify refusing to help almost all couples seeking help in reproducing. A more balanced view would be that being teased at school might make a child unhappy but hardly justifies the claim that it means that overall his life would not be worth living. Where courts have had to decide whether it might be in the best interests of very young children to be allowed to die rather than have life-extending treatment they have set the standards very high: that is, the life has to be very bad for the courts to decide that it would be in the child's best interests to be allowed to die. The outcry at helping the post-menopausal woman to conceive was based on the grounds that the life of the child who may exist as a result of the treatment would not go as well as children born to a younger mother. But that, as I have argued, is not relevant to the question of the best interests of the child who would come to exist were we to help the woman. That child could not exist as the child of a younger woman.

Identity-preserving and identity-affecting actions

There is a fundamental distinction that arises from this discussion: that between an identity-preserving and an identity-affecting action or decision.

An example of an identity-preserving action is when a pregnant woman drinks large amounts of alcohol. The drinking of the alcohol in this example does not affect the identity of the foetus. If the child is subsequently born with some brain damage as a result of the mother's alcohol intake that child has been harmed by the alcohol intake.

An example of an identity-affecting action is when a woman delays reproduction from, for example, 30 to 40 years of age. A different child will be born as a result of her delay. When a doctor chooses to help couple A to conceive, rather than couple B, she is making an identity-affecting decision.

What is the effect of the identity-affecting nature of an act on the morality of that act? This is a question that was first asked in the context of the analysis of fundamental moral theory. It is a question that is becoming of increasing importance to doctors.

The non-identity problem and identity-affecting interventions

Derek Parfit called this issue the non-identity problem. He explains the problem using the example of 'the 14 year old girl'. He writes:

> This girl chooses to have a child. Because she is so young, she gives her child a bad start in life. Though this will have bad effects throughout this child's life, his life will, predictably, be worth living. If this girl had waited for several years, she would have had a different child, to whom she would have given a better start in life.
>
> (p. 358)

> Suppose that we tried to persuade this girl that she ought to wait . . . 'You should think not only of yourself, but also of your child. It will be worse for him if you have him now. If you have him later, you will give him a better start in life.' . . .

> We failed to persuade this girl . . . Were we right to claim that her decision was worse for her child? If she had waited, this particular

child would never have existed. And, despite its bad start, his life is worth living ... 'If someone lives a life that is worth living, is this worse for this person than if he had never existed?' Our answer must be No ... When we see this, do we change our mind about this decision? Do we cease to believe that it would have been better if this girl had waited, so that she could give to her first child a better start in life? ... We cannot claim that this girl's decision was worse for her child. What is the objection to her decision? This question arises because, in different outcomes, different people would be born. I shall therefore call this the *Non-Identity Problem*.

(p. 359)

Parfit's example raises many issues other than the non-identity problem, not least of which is what is in the interests of the girl herself. I want to set these other issues to one side. In the box overleaf, I give some further medical situations in which the non-identity problem arises. In all these cases it can certainly be argued that it would be better if the decision were made that would lead to the birth of whichever child would be likely to have the better life. Such an argument could be based on the idea of maximizing overall welfare. In none of the cases, however, can an argument be based on the interests of the potential child. Nor can it be claimed, whichever decision is made in the three cases, that the child born has been harmed by the decision.

The non-identity issue has an important impact on what doctors should do. Where the doctor aids an act, such as in prescribing during pregnancy a drug that may harm a foetus, then such harm provides a good reason for the doctor to refuse to prescribe the drug even when the woman wants it and it is appropriate treatment. Prescribing this drug is an example of an identity-preserving action. But when the doctor's action is an identity-affecting action that may lead to a child being born with a handicap then there is no child who has been made worse off than she could have otherwise been. In societies that give considerable weight both to patient autonomy and reproductive choice, doctors should not normally override a

Three clinical examples that involve the non-identity problem

1. Preimplantation genetic testing

Hypothetical case 1: 'deafening' an embryo. A couple with a genetic condition causing deafness wish to have a child who is also deaf. This is so that the child is part of the 'deaf community'. The woman becomes pregnant. Genetic testing shows that the foetus does not have the gene causing deafness: it is likely to become a normal child. Suppose that a drug is available that if taken by a pregnant woman will cause a normal foetus to become deaf. It has no other effect and is otherwise completely safe for both embryo and mother. The couple decide that the woman should take this drug in order to ensure that their child is born deaf.

(a) Would the couple be morally wrong to choose to take the drug?

(b) Would a doctor be wrong to prescribe the drug at the couples' request?

(c) If the parents did take the drug and their child were born deaf, would the child have a morally legitimate grievance against the parents, and/or the doctors?

I imagine that most people will answer 'yes' to these three questions. Now consider the following hypothetical case.

Hypothetical case 2: choosing a 'deaf embryo'. A couple with a genetic condition causing deafness wish to have help with conceiving. A number of embryos are created, using IVF (the sperm fertilizes the egg in a laboratory and outside the woman's body, and the fertilized egg is then implanted into the woman's uterus/womb). These are genetically tested to see which have the 'deafness gene'. Embryo A is a genetically normal embryo. Embryo B has the 'deafness gene' but is otherwise genetically normal. The couple choose to have embryo B implanted and subsequently give birth to a deaf child: child B. (If you consider that the embryo has the full moral status of a person, vary the example to involve egg, rather than embryo, selection.)

(a) Are the couple morally wrong to choose, for implantation, embryo B rather than embryo A?
(b) Would doctors be acting wrongly to accede to their request?
(c) Does child B have a morally legitimate grievance against the parents and/or the doctors?

At first sight it seems wrong for the couple to choose to have a deaf child when they could have had a child with normal hearing, and wrong for doctors to allow such a choice. The principal reason why this seems wrong is that such a choice would be harmful to the child. But this is false: it is not harmful to the child because the choice of which embryo to implant is an identity-affecting choice (see text).

2. Delaying pregnancy

A 35-year-old woman hopes in the long run to become a mother, but not yet. She wants to delay pregnancy for another four years until she has finished a degree course. She knows that she is more likely to conceive a child with Down's syndrome if she delays pregnancy. (Down's syndrome is caused by an extra chromosome over the normal number, i.e. 47 rather than 46. Most people with Down's syndrome have some degree of learning difficulty.) She asks her doctor for a prescription for the contraceptive pill. The doctor prescribes the pill for the next three and a half years. After this the woman becomes pregnant and has a child with Down's syndrome. Did the doctor's act, in prescribing the contraceptive pill, harm the child?

3. Treating acne

Acne is a skin condition that typically affects adolescents. It is characterized by spots and small pustules that are distributed over the face. Most adolescents experience mild acne but some suffer a much more severe form. Severe acne, if left untreated, can lead not only to psychological problems but also to permanent facial scarring. Sometimes the only effective treatment for severe acne is a drug called isotretinoin. There is one, very important, unwanted effect of isotretinoin: it may cause foetal damage if a woman is taking the treatment during pregnancy. Children may be born with congenital malformations mainly of facial appearance or of the heart.

Because of the significance of these unwanted effects on a foetus it would normally be considered wrong for a doctor to prescribe isotretinoin to a woman with severe acne known to be pregnant, even if the woman wanted the treatment, because of the harm to the foetus, or at any rate the child that the foetus will become.

What should a doctor do, however, in circumstances where a patient is not pregnant, but might become so while taking the drug? The advice that is given to doctors on this issue is that they should only prescribe the isotretinoin if the woman will reliably delay pregnancy until after she has stopped taking the isotretinoin. In some situations this will require the doctor to prescribe the isotretinoin only in combination with the contraceptive pill.

On this view it is right for a doctor to prescribe isotretinoin to a non-pregnant woman if she will reliably delay pregnancy until after the course of isotretinoin (typically six months to a year); but wrong to prescribe it if she will not reliably delay pregnancy. The intuition is that if she does not delay pregnancy then she has harmed the child, but if she does delay pregnancy then she has not harmed the child. Once again, however, it will be a different child. If she becomes pregnant, and the child is born with a handicap, it cannot be claimed that the child has been harmed as a result of the woman's not delaying pregnancy. For if the woman had delayed pregnancy that child would not have existed at all.

woman's choice in situations where no person is harmed; and in identity-affecting decisions, or acts, no person is harmed (unless the handicap is so severe that the child's life, overall, would not be worth living). Such a conclusion goes against normal intuition. In this case, it seems to me, normal intuition is wrong: it is based on a false metaphysics.

Chapter 5
A tool-box for reasoning

Let me add a certain virile reply recorded by De Quincey (*Writings* XI, 226). Someone flung a glass of wine in the face of a gentleman during a theological or literary debate. The victim did not show any emotion and said to the offender: 'This, sir, is a digression: now, if you please, for the argument.' (The author of that reply, a certain Dr Henderson, died in Oxford around 1787, without leaving us any memory other than those just words: a sufficient and beautiful immortality.)

(J. L. Borges, The Art of Verbal Abuse, 1933)

Medical ethics is, in my view, a questioning and a critically reflective discipline. Doctors, nurses, and other health professionals will normally have good reasons for doing what they do. It would be foolish not to give careful consideration to what experienced practitioners do and think is right. But the role of philosophy is to demand reasons and to subject these reasons to careful critical analysis. Socrates saw himself as an intellectual gad-fly irritating the status quo with awkward questions. Medical practice should be continually improving through subjecting itself to the scrutiny of those twin disciplines, science and philosophy. Science asks: What is the evidence that this is the best treatment? How good is that evidence? What evidence is there for alternative treatments? Philosophy demands reasons for the moral choices made: Is it right to help this single woman to conceive a child using methods of assisted reproduction? Should all attempts be made to prolong the life of this patient using the facilities of intensive care, or should she be allowed to die but in as little distress as possible?

Everyone expects philosophical reasoning to be rigorous, to be logically valid. But what makes philosophy in general, and ethics in particular, so exciting is that providing reasons, and giving arguments, requires not only intellectual rigour but also imagination. Ethics uses many tools of reasoning, but it is not just a question of learning how to use the tools: there is always the possibility of a leap of the imagination – of a different perspective or an interesting comparison that puts the whole question in a new light and takes our thinking forward.

I have already made use of a number of these different tools: logical argument, false arguments, definitions, and the slippery slope argument in Chapter 2; case comparisons, including thought experiments, in Chapters 2 and 3; conceptual analysis and the identification of conceptual distinctions in Chapter 4. Let us examine some of these tools of ethical reasoning in more detail.

The first tool: logic

A valid argument must be logically sound. An argument is a set of reasons supporting a conclusion. A deductive, or logical, argument is a series of statements (called premises) which lead logically to a conclusion. A valid argument is one in which the conclusion follows as a matter of logical necessity from the premises. The conclusion from a valid argument may or may not be true. Near the beginning of Chapter 2, I put forward a logically valid argument in the form of a syllogism but I claimed that the conclusion was false on the grounds that one of the premises was false.

A syllogism is an argument that can be expressed in the form of two propositions, called premises, and a conclusion that results, as a matter of logic, from the premises. There are two main types of valid syllogism.

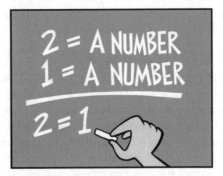

13. Logic is the first tool of argument. But beware false logic.

Valid syllogism – type 1

Premise 1 (P1)   If p then q (If statement p is true then statement q is true)

Premise 2 (P2)   p (i.e. statement p is true)

Conclusion (C)   q (therefore statement q is true)

The technical name for this type of syllogism is *modus ponens*. An example is as follows:

P1   If a foetus is a person it is wrong to kill it

P2   A foetus is a person

C   It is wrong to kill a foetus

Valid syllogism – type 2

Premise 1   If p then q (If statement p is true then statement q is true)

Premise 2   Not q (it is not the case that q is true; q is false)

Conclusion   Not p (therefore statement p is false)

The technical name for this type of syllogism is *modus tollens*. An example is as follows:

P1   If a foetus is a person it is wrong to kill it

P2 It is not wrong to kill a foetus

C   A foetus is not a person

There is one type of invalid, or logically false, argument that people often make. It is worth being on the look-out for this.

An invalid argument in the form of a syllogism

Premise 1	If p then q (If statement p is true then statement q is true)
Premise 2	Not p (i.e. statement p is false)
False Conclusion	Not q (therefore statement q is false)

An example is as follows:

P1 If a foetus is a person it is wrong to kill it

P2 A foetus is not a person

C   It is not wrong to kill a foetus

There may be reasons why it is wrong to kill a foetus other than its being a person.

When you are examining an argument in medical ethics it can be useful to try and boil the argument down to its basic form, as I did in Chapter 2 when discussing what I called 'playing the Nazi card'. This enables the premises to be clearly identified – and examined – and will help expose any fallacy in the argument itself. Medical ethics, and applied philosophy more generally, is concerned with constructing arguments about what we should do, based on premises that we should all accept.

The second tool: conceptual analysis

An important component of valid reasoning is conceptual analysis. There are four types of conceptual analysis: providing a definition; elucidating a concept; making distinctions (splitting); and identifying similarities between two different concepts (lumping). Not that these components can always be kept separate. In

Chapter 2, for example, I provided some definitions for different types of euthanasia. This process of defining is part and parcel of making distinctions; they are not separate activities. The clarification of concepts is a crucial and demanding task in medical ethics. We often use concepts that are unproblematic in most situations but become quite opaque when applied in a new context. An important concept in medicine is that of the best interests of a patient. In both English and US law a doctor is usually obliged to treat a patient in his best interests. If the patient is a young man with appendicitis it is pretty clear that his best interests are served by removing the appendix. It is much less clear what management plan is in the best interests of a man with severe Alzheimer's disease who also has cancer of the bowel. Part of the issue is what factors make up 'best interests' in this situation, and who is to make the judgements. The issue is even more problematic when we are talking about the best interests, or the welfare, of a child who may exist in the future, as we saw in the last chapter.

The third tool: consistency and case comparison

The underlying principle of consistency is that if you conclude that you should make different decisions, or do different things, in two similar situations then you must be able to point to a morally relevant difference between the two situations that accounts for the different decisions. Otherwise you are being inconsistent.

In Chapter 2, I made a comparison between what Dr Cox did (inject potassium chloride) and what many doctors quite legitimately do (inject morphine) in situations similar to that faced by Dr Cox. So why, I asked, should Dr Cox, but not those doctors who inject morphine, face the serious criminal charge of (attempted) murder? Is this inconsistent practice, or is there a morally relevant difference? The obvious difference is that Dr Cox intended that his patient die, whereas those who inject morphine do not intend death although they might foresee it. Whether this distinction between *intending* and *foreseeing* is morally relevant is an issue requiring further analysis.

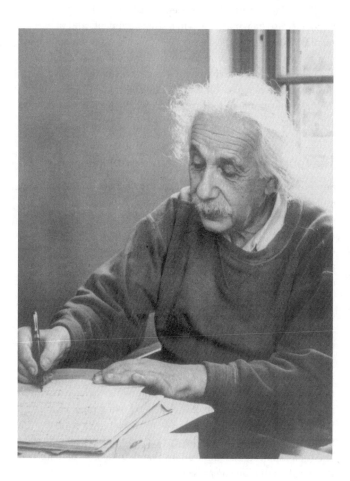

14. Einstein used thought experiments as a tool for the scientific understanding of the universe. Thought experiments are a vital tool in ethics as well.

Thought experiments

The cases used for case comparison, or for examining consistency, may be real or hypothetical, or even unrealistic. Philosophers frequently use imaginary cases in testing arguments and in examining concepts. These are called 'thought experiments' – like many scientific experiments they are designed to test a theory. I have already used several thought experiments in this book. One of the uses of the imagination is in thinking of thought experiments that take the argument forward, or that challenge our routine ways of thinking.

The fourth tool: reasoning from principles

Several books and many articles organize the analysis of medical ethics around four principles and their scope of application (see opposite box). These principles might best be seen as perspectives rather than as the premises of a logical argument. They can act as a useful check that a full range of perspectives has been taken into account. When considering whether or not a doctor should breach a patient's confidentiality, for example, it may be helpful to identify the key issues by examining the situation from the perspective of each principle. This is, however, only the beginning. Further conceptual analysis (e.g. what do we mean by best interests in this situation) and judgement will be needed.

Another form of 'top-down' reasoning is to argue, not from one of the four principles, but from a general moral theory such as utilitarianism. A discussion of such general moral theories is beyond the scope of this book. In essence such top–down reasoning involves identifying a moral theory that you think is generally right and then exploring the implications that that theory would have in the specific situation you are considering.

Reasoning about morality involves, in my view, a continual moving between our moral responses to specific situations (or cases) and our moral theories. Rawls called this process *reflective equilibrium*.

Four principles in medical ethics

1. Respect for patient autonomy

Autonomy (literally self-rule) is the capacity to think, decide, and act on the basis of such thought and decision, freely and independently (Gillon 1986). Respect for patient autonomy requires health professionals (and others, including the patient's family) to help patients to come to their own decisions (e.g. by providing important information) and to respect and follow those decisions (even when the health professional believes that the patient's decision is wrong).

2. Beneficence: the promotion of what is best for the patient

This principle emphasizes the moral importance of doing good to others and, in particular in the medical context, doing good to patients. Following this principle would entail doing what was best for the patient. This raises the question of who should be the judge of what is best for the patient. This principle is often interpreted as focusing on what an objective assessment by a relevant health professional would determine as in the patient's best interests. The patient's own views are captured by the principle of respect for patient autonomy.

The two principles conflict when a competent patient chooses a course of action which is not in his or her best interests.

3. Non-maleficence: avoiding harm

This principle is the other side of the coin of the principle of beneficence. It states that we should not harm patients. In most situations this principle does not add anything useful to the principle of beneficence. The main reason for retaining the principle of non-maleficence is that it is generally thought that we have a prima-facie duty not to harm anyone, whereas we owe a duty of beneficence to a limited number of people only.

4. Justice

There are four components to this principle: distributive justice; respect for the law; rights; and retributive justice.

With regard to distributive justice: first, patients in similar situations should normally have access to the same health care; and second, in determining what level of health care should be available for one set of patients we must take into account the effect of such a use of resources on other patients. In other words, we must try to distribute our limited resources (time, money, intensive care beds) fairly.

The second component of justice is whether the fact that some act is, or is not, against the law is of moral relevance. Whilst many people take the view that it may, in some situations, be morally right to break the law, nevertheless if laws are made through a reasonable democratic process they have moral force.

The types and status of rights are much disputed. The fundamental idea is that if a person has a right it gives her a special advantage – a safeguard so that her right is respected even if the overall social good is thereby diminished.

'Retributive' justice concerns the fitting of the punishment to the crime. In the medical context this issue is sometimes raised when a person with mental disorder commits a crime.

During the process both the theories and the beliefs about individual situations can undergo revision. When there is lack of agreement between theory and our intuitions about individual cases, there is no algorithm, or computer program, that can tell us which or what we must change. That has to be a matter of judgement.

Spotting fallacies in reasoning

Logicians like to spot, and name, fallacious arguments, rather
as ornithologists spot birds. We came across the *argumentum
ad hominem* in Chapter 2. Spotting fallacies is a useful
exercise in medical ethics because it helps us to see through
a rhetorically powerful but ultimately false argument. Here
are two of my favourite fallacies named and defined by
Flew (1989).

The No-True Scotsman Move

> Someone says: 'No Scotsman would beat his wife to a shapeless pulp
> with a blunt instrument'. He is confronted with a falsifying instance:
> 'Mr Angus McSporran did just that'. Instead of withdrawing, or at
> least qualifying, the too rash original claim our patriot insists: 'Well,
> no true Scotsman would do such a thing!'

What seems to be a statement of fact (an empirical claim) is made
impervious to counter-examples by adapting the meaning of the
words so that the statement becomes true by definition and empty
of any empirical content.

The Ten-Leaky-Buckets Tactic

This is

> presenting a series of severally unsound arguments as if their
> mere conjunction might render them collectively valid: something
> that needs to be distinguished carefully from the accumulation of
> evidence, where every item possesses some weight in its own
> right.

Nature and Playing God

There are two arguments that we met in Chapter 2 and that I
promised to consider in more detail: the argument from Nature and
the argument from Playing God.

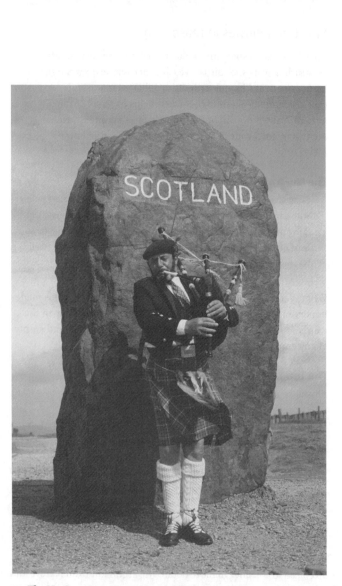

15. The No-True Scotsman Move: a fallacy in argument.

The argument from Nature

Stated baldly the argument from Nature boils down to the assertion: this is not natural, therefore this is morally wrong. The argument has been used against homosexuality, and it is often brought out in the context of medical ethics, not only when considering euthanasia but also when discussing possibilities arising from modern reproductive technology and genetics. The argument is problematic in at least three ways. First, it is not entirely clear what it means to say that something is unnatural. If about 10 per cent of humans are predominantly homosexual, and homosexual behaviour is seen in other species, what is meant by saying that homosexuality is unnatural? Second, it seems quite unclear why it follows from the fact that something is unnatural, that it is morally wrong. What kind of reason could be given in support of this? Third, there are an enormous number of counter-examples, not least from medical practice itself, to the claim that what is unnatural is morally wrong. The life of a child with meningitis may be saved by antibiotics and intensive care. Neither treatment is 'natural' by any meaning that can be given to that term. Perhaps it is wrong to help couples to have babies using in-vitro fertilization (IVF) but, if it is wrong, that cannot be on the grounds that IVF is unnatural.

The argument from Playing God

The argument from Playing God can also be stated baldly as: this act is morally wrong because it is playing God. The argument is problematic in ways analogous to the problem with the argument from Nature. What criteria can be used to distinguish between our carrying out God's will, and our usurping his role? Which of the following is playing God: providing IVF; withdrawing life support; injecting antibiotics; transplanting a kidney? It seems to me that we have first to decide which acts are right or wrong before we can determine those that might be described as playing God. The concept of Playing God is therefore of no help in determining what it is right to do.

The slippery slope argument

I want finally, in this chapter on methods of reasoning, to turn to
the slippery slope argument. This is often used in medical ethics.
The core of the argument is that once you accept one particular
position then it will be extremely difficult, or indeed impossible, not
to accept more and more extreme positions. If you do not want to
accept the more extreme positions you must not accept the original,
less extreme position.

One example of the use of such an argument is against the practice
of voluntary active euthanasia as I raised briefly in Chapter 2.
Suppose, for example, that a supporter of voluntary active
euthanasia gave an example of a situation when it seemed plausible
to agree that euthanasia, in that situation, is acceptable. The case of
mercy killing carried out by Dr Cox (p. 13) might be such an
example. The slippery slope argument could be used against killing
the patient, not on the grounds that it would be wrong as a matter of
principle in this case, but on the grounds that allowing killing in
this case would inevitably lead to allowing killing in situations
where it would be wrong.

The main counter to the slippery slope argument is to claim that a
barrier can be placed part way down the slope so that in stepping
onto the top of the slope we will not inevitably slide to the bottom –
but only as far as the barrier.

There are two types of slippery slope argument: a logical type and
an empirical type.

The logical type of slippery slope argument and the sorites paradox

The logical type of slippery slope argument can be seen as
consisting in three steps:

Step 1: As a matter of logic, if you accept the (apparently reasonable) proposition, p, then you must also accept the closely related proposition, q. Similarly, if you accept q you must accept proposition r, and so on through propositions s, t, etc. The propositions p, q, r, s, t, etc. form a series of related propositions such that adjacent propositions are more similar to each other than those further apart in the series.

Step 2: This involves showing, or gaining agreement from the other side in the argument, that at some stage in this series the propositions become clearly unacceptable, or false.

Step 3: This involves applying formal logic (*modus tollens*) to conclude that since one of the later propositions (e.g. proposition t) is false, it follows that the first proposition (p) is false.

In summary, step 1 is to establish the premise: *if p then t*. Step 2 is to establish the premise: *t is false*. Step 3 is to point out that from these premises it follows, logically, that *p is false*.

It is the first step in the argument that is special about slippery slopes. The crucial component in the argument is to establish a series of propositions such that adjacent members of the series are so close that there can be no reasonable grounds for holding one proposition true (or false) and its adjacent proposition(s) false (or true).

This logical form of slippery slope argument is related closely to a class of paradoxes known as the 'sorites paradoxes' first identified by the ancient Greeks (purportedly by Eubulides – see Priest 2000).

The name 'sorites' comes from the Greek 'soros', meaning a heap. An early example of this type of paradox involved arguing that one grain of sand does not make a heap, and adding one grain of sand to something that is not a heap will not make a heap, so you can never have a heap of sand.

These types of paradox arise because many (perhaps most) of the concepts we use have a certain vagueness: if a concept applies to one object then the concept will still apply if there is a very small change in that object. But a casual observation of children playing on the beach will show that heaps of sand do exist and that the logical form of slippery slope argument is unsound. Proposition t may be false while proposition p is true. There are three possible responses to a slippery slope argument.

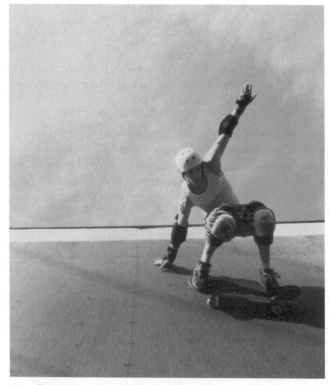

16. A slippery slope may be converted to a stairway.

1. To argue that each small change makes a small, if imperceptible, moral difference (like each grain of sand).

2. To draw the line, or place a barrier, at some stage along the slope. The precise drawing of the line is arbitrary; but it is not arbitrary that a line is drawn. In order to ensure clear policy (and clear laws) it is often sensible to draw precise lines even though the underlying concepts and moral values change more gradually.

3. A third response, which is not always appropriate, is to place a barrier at a position that is not arbitrary but is justified for some principled reason. In the case of euthanasia a proponent might argue that there is a difference between voluntary active euthanasia and other types, such as non-voluntary active euthanasia. In accepting the possibility of voluntary active euthanasia one does not have to slide into accepting non-voluntary, or involuntary, active euthanasia: the logical relationships are more like a stairway than a slippery slope.

The empirical form of slippery slope argument

The second form of slippery slope argument is empirical, or 'in practice', not logical. An opponent of voluntary active euthanasia might argue that if we allow doctors to carry out such euthanasia, then, as a matter of fact, in the real world, this will lead to non-voluntary euthanasia (or beyond). Such an opponent might accept that there is no logical reason to slip from the one to the other, but that in practice such slippage will occur. Therefore we should, as a matter of policy not legitimate voluntary active euthanasia even if such euthanasia is not, in principle, wrong.

This empirical form of argument depends on making assumptions about how the world actually is and therefore raises the question of how compelling is the evidence for such assumptions. What will in practice happen will often depend on how precisely the policy is worded, or enforced. It may be possible to prevent slipping down the slope by putting up a barrier; or by careful articulation of the circumstances under which an action is, or is not, legitimate.

In this chapter I have stepped back from specific issues in medical ethics in order to reflect on some of the tools of reasoning. I will now return to issues and in the next chapter I will claim that the law is unjust in the way it deals with people who are mentally ill. I will start with the claim that the law is inconsistent.

Chapter 6
Inconsistencies about madness

43rd day of April in the year 2000: Today we celebrate a most illustrious event! Spain has a king. He has been found. I am this king ... Now everything has been revealed to me. I see it all as clearly as my own hand. But before this, I don't know why, before I seemed to see everything through some sort of fog. I think this all can be explained by the ridiculous idea people have that the brain is in the head. Nothing of the kind: it is carried by the wind from the direction of the Caspian Sea.

(Gogol, *Diary of a Madman*, 1835)

In 1851 Dr Samuel Cartwright published an article in the *New Orleans Medical and Surgical Journal* describing the mental illness of drapetomania (quoted in Reznek, 1987). This was an illness from which Negro slaves suffered: it was manifest by a tendency to run away from their white masters.

In 1952 the first edition of the *US Diagnostic and Statistical Manual of Mental Disorders* was published. This is the main US classification of mental illness. Homosexuality was listed as a mental disorder and its status was confirmed in the second edition of the manual in 1968. In 1973 there was debate in the American Psychiatric Association as to the medical status of homosexuality. By a small majority the Association voted to remove homosexuality from the list of mental disorders.

The classificatory system of disease that is used in most of Europe, including the UK, is the International Classification of Diseases. The current edition includes fetishism as a mental disorder. This is described as:

> Reliance on some non-living object as stimulus for sexual arousal and sexual gratification. Many fetishes are extensions of the human body, such as articles of clothing or footwear. Other common examples are characterised by some particular texture such as rubber, plastic or leather.

The diagnosis of fetishism can be made if the person experiences recurrent intense sexual urges and fantasies involving such objects, if he acts on these, if the preference has been present for more than six months, and if the object is the most important source of sexual stimulation. Will fetishism still be classified as a mental disorder in 20 years' time?

The social and ethical values that lie behind the diagnosis and classification of mental disorders have been under attack since the anti-psychiatry movement in the 1960s. What we count as 'healthy' or 'unhealthy' sometimes reflects our value commitments, and these can, and should, be challenged. Although the question of what is a mental illness can raise deep and difficult problems, I am going to put these to one side. Some conditions, such as schizophrenia, do render people out of touch with reality, and cause suffering, to such an extent that I will take for granted that these conditions are the proper concern of the medical specialty of psychiatry. What I want to examine in this chapter are the different standards used in enforcing treatment and secure accommodation for those with and without mental disorder. I will argue that those with mental disorder are subject to a double injustice.

Most Western countries have special legislation to allow patients with mental disorder to be kept in hospital, and treated, against

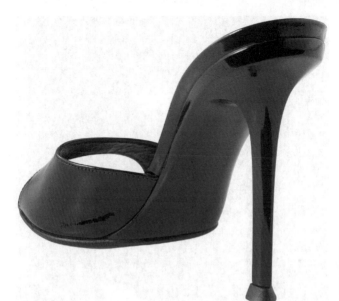

17. Not long ago homosexuality was classified as a mental illness. Fetishism still is.

their will. Such legislation typically addresses two issues: first, when can treatment be imposed on patients with mental illness, for their own sake, in situations where they are refusing treatment; and second, how can society be protected from potentially dangerous people with mental illness? I believe it is mistaken to attempt to do these two different things within one body of legislation.

Crime and mental illness

It is the criminal law that deals mainly with the question of public protection. It is problematic, however, to treat mentally ill people as criminals when their dangerous and illegal behaviour is a result of mental illness. In English law, as well as in the law of many other

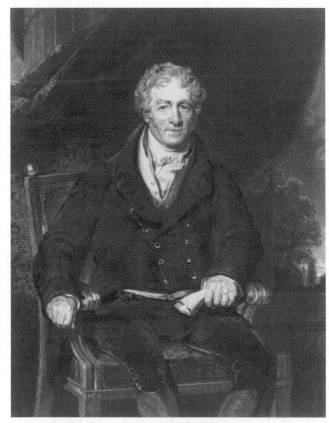

18. An attempt to assassinate the British Prime Minister, Sir Robert Peel, in 1843, led to the establishment of the legal rules for determining when a person is not guilty of a crime on grounds of insanity.

countries, for a person to be found guilty of a crime two points have to be proven: that it was this person who carried out the relevant act; and that this person had the state of mind necessary to be held responsible for that act. The first aspect is known as the *actus reus* ('guilty act') and the second as the *mens rea* ('guilty mind'). The precise *mens rea* required varies from crime to crime. For example, to be guilty of *murder* a person must have had 'specific intent', i.e. must have had the intention to kill (or cause serious physical harm to) the victim. To be found guilty of *manslaughter* it is necessary only to establish that the person showed gross negligence.

It is a long-established liberal principle that a person who suffers from a mental illness may be found 'not guilty', even though he committed a criminal act, on the grounds that he should not be held responsible for his behaviour, because of the illness. Crudely put: the person's body committed the act, but the person's mind did not commit the crime.

A key English case was that of Daniel McNaughten who, like Shakespeare, spelt his name in many different ways. McNaughten suffered delusional beliefs, including the belief that the British Tory Party was behind a plot to kill him. He decided to kill its leader, Sir Robert Peel. In 1843 he shot Peel's secretary, Edward Drummond, but was prevented from firing a second shot. McNaughten was acquitted of murder on the grounds of insanity and was sent to a secure psychiatric hospital (the Bethlem hospital in South London, which is the origin of the word *bedlam*). The acquittal caused public outrage. The House of Lords asked the judges to draw up rules (now known as the McNaughten rules) for determining when someone should be considered 'not guilty' on grounds of insanity.

Protecting society from dangerous people

A person without mental disorder who commits a violent crime of sufficient gravity is typically sent to prison. There are a number of reasons for sending such a person to prison. One reason is as retribution: he deserves to be punished. Another reason is to protect society.

There are two crucial liberal principles that are incorporated into criminal law – and are part of the European law on human rights:

1. A person who has not (yet) committed a crime cannot be detained on the grounds that it is expected that he will commit a crime.
2. A person must be allowed back into the community once he has served his prison sentence, although some crimes may attract a life sentence.

These two principles apply, however, only to those who do not suffer a mental disorder. If you have committed a violent act as a result of mental illness you can be detained in a psychiatric hospital as long as it is thought that you pose sufficient risk to others. This may well be much longer than a mentally healthy criminal would have been detained in prison for a similar violent act. Indeed you may be so detained even if you have not yet committed a violent act. I will use the term 'preventive detention' to refer to keeping someone in a secure environment (prison or a secure psychiatric hospital) on grounds of protection of others in one, or both, of the following situations: when the person has not (yet) committed a violent act; and when he has committed such an act and been in a secure environment for the length of the prison sentence appropriate to the act. The two liberal principles stated above can now be rewritten as: 'A person should not be preventively detained'. What worries me is that this applies to those without mental disorder but not to those with mental disorder. And that is unfair.

There is, of course, an important issue of public policy as to how society should protect itself against people who pose significant risk of harm to others. In the UK this is a particularly live issue in the context of those who pose a threat to children. The argument I want to make is an argument about consistency. If two people, A, who is mentally ill, and B, who is not mentally ill, pose the same risk of harm to others, then, if it is right to preventively detain A (on grounds of this risk of harm) it is right to do so to B. Conversely if it is wrong to preventively detain B (as European legislation states) then it is wrong to detain A. Otherwise we are discriminating against the mentally ill.

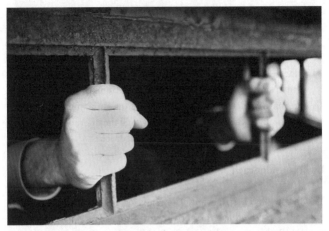

19. A criminal who has served his sentence must be released from prison even if he remains dangerous. A mentally disordered patient who remains dangerous may be kept locked up forever. Is this fair?

Are there any reasons that justify such apparent discrimination? I can think of four possible reasons, but none, in my opinion, justifies a different approach to preventive detention.

1. The mentally ill person is more dangerous.
2. The assessment of risk of harm is more certain in the case of those with mental illness.
3. It may be the case that prolonging detention in hospital will lead to further improvement in the mental illness and further reduction in risk of harm to others. It would be silly to release the patient from the secure psychiatric hospital when a further period in hospital would reduce risk.
4. The final reason depends on a distinction being made between what a person wants when mentally ill, and what the person would want if cured of the mental illness. It is typically the case that those mentally ill patients who are preventively detained remain chronically ill. That is why they remain at risk of harming others, and why they continue to be detained. It is possible, at least in

theory, to distinguish between what the ill person wants, and what the person might have wanted if well – even though he remains ill. It might be argued that his genuine wishes are those he would have when well. Since the danger he poses to others is due to the mental illness, it might reasonably be expected that if he were well he would say that he would like, when ill and a danger to others, to be preventively detained. Thus respecting the authentic wishes and autonomy of the person when well would mean preventively detaining the person when ill (and dangerous).

I will consider each of these four reasons in turn.

The first reason is irrelevant. The situation I am considering is where the two people – the person with, and the person without, the mental illness – pose the same risk of harm to others.

The second reason might provide weak grounds for a difference in approach if it were true; but it is not. Assessment of risk of harm to others is notoriously difficult whether we are dealing with mentally disordered people or not. In any case the point at issue is whether risk of harm justifies preventive detention. The level of uncertainty over the estimation of risk might alter the threshold but not the principle of preventive detention.

The third reason does not provide grounds for treating those with mental illness differently from those without. In both cases a detained person might pose less of a risk of harm to others if further detained. If this continuing reduction in risk gives grounds for preventive detention in those with mental illness then it also provides grounds for preventive detention of those without. I don't believe, however, that it gives good grounds in either case. If preventive detention is to be justified then it should be on the grounds of the risk of harm to others. If two people pose similar risks then they should be treated similarly.

The fourth reason provides the best argument but even this is unconvincing. The mentally disordered people we are talking about tend to be either those with chronic mental illness or personality disorder. There is unlikely to be good evidence that the person's 'authentic wishes' would be to continue to be detained. In the absence of such evidence it seems highly dubious to keep the person locked up on the grounds of respecting his autonomy.

I conclude that if we think it right for society to lock away mentally ill people who present a certain level of risk of harm to others then we should do the same for those who are not mentally ill. Conversely if we think preventive detention is an unacceptable infringement of human rights in the case of people without mental illness, it is an unacceptable infringement of human rights for those with mental illness. I leave open which way we ought to go. The point I want to make is that the current position is untenable, because inconsistent and unjust.

Enforcing treatment for the sake of the mentally ill person

I wrote at the beginning of this chapter that those with mental disorder are subject to a double injustice. They are discriminated against not only for the protection of others but also for the protection of themselves. It is a long-standing principle in medical ethics and law that those who are ill may refuse what their doctors and others believe is beneficial treatment. A classic example is when a Jehovah's Witness refuses blood transfusion even when she is likely to die without the transfusion. It is a principle in many legal systems that a competent adult has a right to refuse any, even life-saving, treatment. This principle applies to the treatment of physical illness. It does not apply however in many countries to those with mental illness. Take the case of England, where it is the Mental Health Act that governs the compulsory treatment of patients with mental disorder.

Under the English Mental Health Act there are three criteria that need to be met in order for a patient to be detained in hospital for treatment:

(1) he should suffer from a mental disorder;
(2) his mental disorder is 'of a nature or degree which makes it appropriate to receive medical treatment in a hospital';
(3) the admission for treatment 'is necessary for the health or safety of the patient or for the protection of other persons'.

I have already considered the inequities inherent when considering the protection of others. I want now to consider the 'health and safety' of the person himself.

What is of note about the Mental Health Act is that a person who has a mental disorder may be treated for his mental disorder despite refusal even if he is competent to give or refuse consent. A competent person with a mental illness can be treated against his will if others (such as a psychiatrist and social worker) think it is appropriate. This is unjust unless anyone with a mental disorder is *ipso facto* not competent to refuse treatment. But this is not the case. The question of whether someone has a mental disorder is a question left mainly to doctors and it covers many psychological problems which cause distress. Some people with a mental disorder will lack decision-making capacity. Some won't.

The issue came under legal scrutiny in England in the case of *B* v *Croydon District Health Authority* (1994). This concerned a 24-year-old woman who had been admitted to psychiatric hospital with a diagnosis of borderline personality disorder. She had a history of self-harm. She was compulsorily detained under the Mental Health Act following her behaviour of trying to cut and hurt herself. In hospital she was prevented from such harmful behaviour, but her response was to virtually stop eating and as a result her weight fell to dangerously low levels. By May 1994 her weight was only 32 kilos and her doctor thought that she would die within a few months if she continued to behave as she was doing.

Her doctors wanted to tube feed her in order to prevent her death. She was granted an injunction to prevent this until the case could come to a full legal hearing. Although by the time the case came to a full hearing she was eating, the High Court considered the question of whether tube feeding would have been lawful.

At the High Court the following points were decided: (1) she was found to have the capacity to refuse treatment; but (2) she had a mental disorder, and therefore, despite having the capacity to refuse treatment, she could be treated compulsorily under the Mental Health Act. This was because it was held that she had a mental disorder of a nature and degree that made it appropriate to receive medical treatment in hospital, and that such admission was necessary for her health and safety.

Again it is the different standards being applied to those with mental disorder, compared to those without, that trouble me. It may be right to impose life-saving treatment on a patient who is refusing, and who is competent to refuse, treatment or it may be wrong. But what does not seem right is to change the answer depending on whether the person has a mental disorder. Of course many mental disorders interfere with competence to refuse treatment. Perhaps the High Court was wrong to decide that B had capacity to refuse treatment. We may need to deepen our understanding of how and when mental disorder interferes with such capacity. But what seems unacceptable to me is to bypass this issue altogether and to treat all those with mental disorder paternalistically, while allowing those without mental disorder the freedom to refuse treatment. To do so is to discriminate, once again, against those suffering from a mental illness.

Chapter 7

How modern genetics is testing traditional confidentiality

What a prodigious thing it is that within the drop of semen which brings us forth there are stamped the characteristics not only of the bodily form of our forefathers but of their ways of thinking and their slant of mind. Where can that drop of fluid lodge such an infinite number of Forms? . . . We can assume that it is to my father that I owe my propensity to the stone, for he died dreadfully afflicted by a large stone in the bladder . . . Now I was born twenty-five years . . . before he fell ill . . . During all that time where did that propensity for this affliction lie a-brooding? When his own illness was still so far off, how did that little piece of his own substance which went to make me manage to transmit so marked a characteristic to me? And how was it so hidden that I only began to be aware of it forty-five years later . . . ?

(Montaigne, 'On the Resemblance of Children to their Fathers')

The fifth metacarpal is the bone that runs along the edge of the palm of the hand between the wrist and the base of the little finger. A fracture to this bone near to the knuckle can result in one way only: from punching someone or something with a clenched fist. Patients, of course, may not like to admit this; but the fracture discloses the truth.

Modern genetics, increasingly, is able both to reveal the past and to foretell the future. And it goes further. A genetic test from one

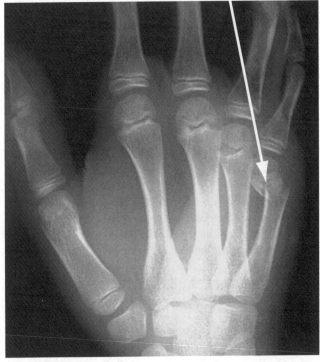

Fracture of
fifth metacarpal

20. A secret revealed. What is the only cause of a fracture, close to the knuckle, of the fifth metacarpal?

person can provide information about a relative. This was possible to a limited extent before modern genetics. What is new is the extent to which these possibilities can be realized; and this extent is forcing us to rethink medical confidentiality.

Case 1: Genetic tests reveal secrets of paternity

Let me start with the revealing of secrets. Here is a realistic case from a modern genetics service reported in *The Lancet*.

John and Sarah attend the genetics clinic after the diagnosis of an autosomal recessive condition in their newborn baby. The disorder is severe and debilitating and there is a high chance that the child will die in the first year. The gene for this disorder has just been mapped and there is a possibility that prenatal diagnosis would be possible in a future pregnancy. John and Sarah give their consent for a blood sample to be taken for DNA extraction, from themselves and their affected child.

At the first meeting with the geneticist the couple are told that the chance of any of their future children having the condition is 25 per cent (see Figure 21). This is correct on the assumption that John was the biological father of Sarah's newborn baby.

Molecular analyses of the DNA samples, however, reveal that John is not the father of the child. One implication of this is that any future baby, who is the biological child of John and Sarah, is very unlikely indeed to have the debilitating condition. This is because

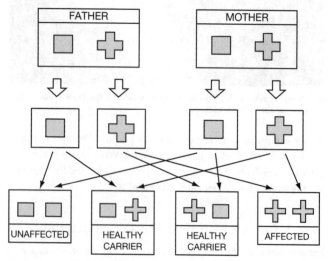

21. **Autosomal recessive inheritance.**

only about one in 1,000 people have the recessive gene. John will almost certainly have the normal gene, and this will prevent his children from having the condition.

Should the geneticist disclose, to John, the finding that John is not the father of the newborn baby?

One important US report recommends disclosure to both partners in situations like this. But this report stands alone in preferring an honest and open approach. The influential Committee on Assessing Genetics Risks at the Institute of Medicine in the US recommends that in cases like these only the woman should be told and that: 'Genetic testing should not be used in ways that disrupt families'. Most surveys suggest that most geneticists support this latter approach, both in the US and Europe. A cross-cultural comparison in 1990 argued that 'Protection of the mother's confidentiality over rides disclosure of true paternity'.

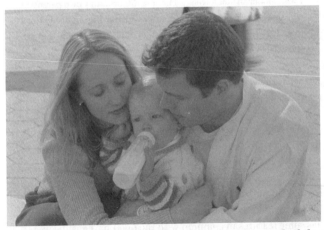

22. **DNA testing shows that, unknown to him, the man is not the father of the baby. What should the genetic counsellor tell him?** (Posed by models.)

Many geneticists would be prepared to tell a lie or fudge the issue, for example by claiming that the child with the condition has the condition as a result of a new mutation, rather than being honest with their patient. A survey of patients, as opposed to doctors, carried out in the US, suggested that three-quarters thought that the doctor ought to tell the husband that he is not the father of the child, at least if he asked directly. The majority of those in that survey were women.

Medical confidentiality

Hippocrates, known as the Father of Medicine, was born on the Greek island of Cos in about 460 BC. The Hippocratic Oath is one of the earliest known sets of professional guidelines for doctors. Some of the guidelines now seem dated. It is unlikely that the medical students whom I teach would see their obligation to me as quite so significant as Hippocrates' Oath would require.

> I will honour the man who teaches me this art as my own parents; I will share my living with him and provide for him in need; I will treat his children as my own brothers and teach them this art, should they wish to learn it, without charge or stipulation . . .

But what the Oath says about confidentiality is much more relevant:

> Whatever I may see or learn about people in the course of my work or in my private life which should not be disclosed I will keep to myself and treat in complete confidence . . .

In order to pursue the question of the limits of confidentiality I want to make a case comparison: to consider a case that has some features in common with the one I have just been discussing, but where it is perhaps clearer what a doctor ought to do.

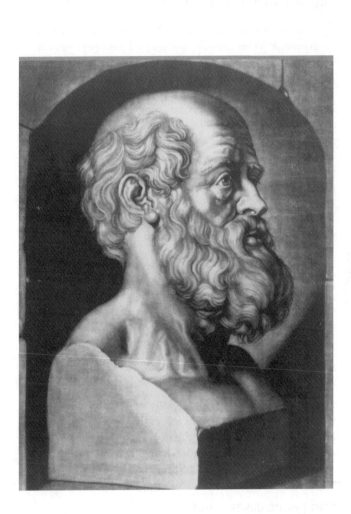

23. Hippocrates, born *c.*460 BC, gives his name to the Hippocratic Oath. This is the origin of medical confidentiality but how should it be interpreted in the era of modern genetics?

Case 2: Paternity revealed by the mother

> . . . following a healthy pregnancy and birth Mary visits her general
> practitioner for her routine 6-week postnatal visit. Mary's husband,
> Peter, is registered with the same GP. During the consultation Mary
> reveals that Peter is not the father of her child.

In a case like this it would be widely accepted that the doctor
should not breach the confidentiality of Mary. Doctors, and other
professionals, have to take professional guidelines seriously into
account when deciding what to do. There would need to be very
good reasons why an individual doctor would go against his
professional guidelines.

The General Medical Council is the professional body for UK
doctors. Its guidelines state:

Medical Ethics

> Disclosure of personal information without consent may be justified
> where failure to do so may expose the patient or others to risk of
> death or serious harm. Where third parties are exposed to a risk so
> serious that it outweighs the patient's privacy interest, you should
> seek consent to disclosure where practicable. If it is not practicable,
> you should disclose information promptly to an appropriate person
> or authority. You should generally inform the patient before
> disclosing the information.

In applying such guidelines to a particular situation some
interpretation is needed. In this case such interpretation seems
relatively straightforward. The harm of not telling Peter does not
amount to 'risk of death or serious harm'. The doctor, therefore,
should not breach Mary's confidentiality.

Comparing cases 1 and 2

If the doctor should not breach confidentiality in case 2, does it
follow that the geneticist should keep quiet about the question of
paternity in case 1?

There are important differences between the two cases. In case 1, the fact of non-paternity was discovered as a result of tests for which both John and Sarah gave consent. In case 2 this fact was revealed only by Mary. In case 1, John and Sarah came to the geneticist together to discuss an issue of joint concern. The information concerning paternity is directly relevant to the issue about which John and Sarah came jointly to see the geneticist. Informing Sarah alone does not respect John's interest in knowing the information.

The foundations of medical confidentiality

The case comparison may leave us in doubt about what the geneticist should do in case 1. Consideration of case 2 provides some reasons why the geneticist should keep information about paternity secret from John. But case 2 differs from case 1 in some important respects that might make all the difference.

Perhaps we can be helped by going back to theory and asking what are the fundamental reasons why maintaining medical confidentiality is important. The three most commonly given answers to this question are: respect for patient autonomy; to keep an implied promise; and to bring about the best consequences.

Respect for the right to privacy

An important principle in medical ethics is respect for patient autonomy (p. 65). This principle emphasizes the patient's right to have control over his own life. This principle implies that a person has the right, by and large, to decide who should have access to information about himself – i.e. a right to privacy. On this view the patient who reveals information about himself to the doctor has the right to determine who else, if anyone, should know that information. That is why the doctor should not normally pass that information on to a third party without the patient's permission.

Implied promise

Some argue that the relationship between doctor and patient has elements of an implied contract. One of these elements is that the doctor, by implication, promises not to breach patient confidentiality. Thus patients may reasonably believe that when they come to their doctors there is an understanding that what they say will be kept confidential. On this view, the reason why a doctor should not breach confidentiality is because to do so would involve breaking a promise.

Best consequences

One of the major theories in moral philosophy claims that the right action in any situation is the one that has the best consequences. On this view, it is important that doctors maintain confidentiality because so doing leads to the best consequences. Only if doctors are strict in maintaining confidentiality will patients trust them. And such trust is vital if patients are to seek and obtain the necessary help from doctors.

Do these theories help us in answering the question: should the geneticist tell John that he is not the father of the newborn baby?

The theory of respect for autonomy is ambiguous when we try to apply it to case 1. It all depends on whose autonomy we focus. John's autonomy is respected by telling John; Sarah's by keeping it secret from John (unless Sarah gives permission to tell John).

The implied promise theory is similarly problematic. In normal clinical practice, as exemplified by case 2, it is clear that the patient (Mary) can expect the doctor to respect her confidentiality. But it is not so clear what the implied elements of the 'contract' are in case 1. John might reasonably expect that all information relevant to future reproductive choices will be shared openly with both him and his wife.

A consequentialist account certainly gives reasons for why the doctor should not breach confidentiality on the grounds of the possible deleterious effect on the family. This is the main reason why most geneticists would not tell John that he is not the biological father of Sarah's child. But it is not entirely clear that the consequences of keeping John ignorant are better than informing him of the truth. Is it right that Sarah needs to be protected from the consequences of her act and will it be better for the family if this remains a secret? This is an example of a major practical problem with consequentialism: even if you think that consequentialism is the right moral theory, it is often impossible to determine with sufficient degree of certainty what the various consequences of different courses of action are likely to be.

It seems that returning to the fundamental theory of what underpins the moral importance of confidentiality has been of no more help than case comparison. We remain uncertain whether the doctor should tell John that he is not the biological father of Sarah's child. The difficulty, I believe, is that we have been focusing on the wrong aspect of the problem. The key question is not whether there are sufficient grounds, in terms of John's interests, for breaching Sarah's confidentiality. The question is whether the information that the newborn baby is not, contrary to John's current belief, his biological baby, is as much 'his information' as Sarah's. Whose information is it? Let us examine this question through the lens of a further case.

Whose information is it? Case 3: Secrets and sisters

A four year old boy has been diagnosed with Duchenne Muscular Dystrophy (DMD) . . . DMD is a severe, debilitating and progressive muscle-wasting disease in which children become wheelchair-bound by their early teens and usually die in their twenties. It is an X-linked recessive condition and whilst it is carried by girls it is only . . . boys who are affected. The boy's mother, Helen, is shown to be a carrier for the mutation. Women who are carriers do not show symptoms of the condition, but half of their sons will inherit it from them and will be affected.

Helen has a sister, Penelope, who is ten weeks pregnant. Penelope's obstetrician referred her to the genetics team after she told him that her nephew had speech and development delay. She told him that although she was not close to her sister and had not discussed it with her, she was concerned about the implications for her own pregnancy. In her discussions with the clinical geneticist (who did not know at this stage that both sisters were patients in the same clinic) Penelope made it clear that she would consider terminating a pregnancy if she knew that the fetus was affected with a serious inherited condition. Speech and development delay are features of a range of conditions and would not of themselves indicate carrier-testing for DMD. In addition, because the DMD gene is large and there are a number of possible mutations, testing without information about which mutation is responsible for the nephew's condition is unlikely to be informative.

At her next meeting with her clinical geneticist, Helen says that she knows that her sister is pregnant and that she understands that the pregnancy could be affected. She also says that she has not discussed this with her sister, partly because they don't really get on, but also because she suspects that if her sister were to find out, and if the fetus turned out to be affected, she would terminate the pregnancy. Helen feels very strongly that this would be wrong. She knows that her sister does not share her views, but Helen says she has thought long and hard about the issues and has decided that she wants her test results and information about her son to remain confidential.

(Parker and Lucassen, *Lancet*, 357 (2001))

I want to put aside the question of whether Penelope should or should not have a termination if her foetus carried the gene. Parker and Lucassen propose two models: the personal account model and the joint account model.

The personal account model

The personal account model is the conventional view of medical confidentiality. On this view the information about Helen's genetic state – as a carrier of Duchenne's muscular dystrophy – 'belongs' to Helen, and Helen alone. Respect for such confidentiality is important. It has, however, long been recognized that there are limits to such confidentiality, as has already been highlighted by the GMC guidelines quoted above. But these limits are the exception. On this view the key question is whether the foreseeable harms to Penelope if the information is not disclosed are sufficiently serious to justify breaching Helen's confidentiality.

The joint account model

On the joint account model, genetic information, like information about a joint bank account, is shared by more than one person. Helen's request is not about the appropriate limits of confidentiality – it would be analogous to asking the bank manager not to reveal information about a joint account to the other account holders. On this view genetic information should be seen in a completely different way from most medical information. It is information that should be available to all 'account holders' – i.e. to all (close) genetically related family members. That is, unless there are good reasons to withhold the information.

These two models see the onus of proof, with respect to sharing information, in opposite ways. On the conventional, personal account, model we ask: are the harms to Penelope so great that they override Helen's right to confidentiality? On the joint account model the genetic information, although obtained from Helen's blood and medical history, 'belongs' to the family. Penelope has a right to such information as it is key information to help her to know important aspects of her genetic make-up. There would need to be a very good reason, in terms of Helen's interests, to justify denying Penelope access to the genetic test for DMD.

Helen knows something not only about herself and her son but also about Penelope and her unborn child. Helen knows that Penelope's foetus has a significant chance of suffering from DMD; but Penelope does not know this. This asymmetry of knowledge is unfair to Penelope. The personal account model fails to take this fact into account.

Genetic information challenges the individualistic nature of many of the moral assumptions made in discussions of medical ethics in both Northern Europe and North America. Perhaps the cases we have been considering raise a deeper issue about medical confidentiality in some other settings. We are interconnected, both biologically and socially. No man is an island, entire of itself. Indeed our connections with each other extend not only to our close genetic relatives but across the globe, as we shall see in the next chapter.

Chapter 8
Is medical research the new imperialism?

> ... a kind, forgiving, charitable, pleasant time; the only time I
> know of, in the long calendar of the year, when men and women
> seem by one consent to open their shut-up hearts freely, and to
> think of people below them as if they really were fellow-passengers
> to the grave, and not another race of creatures bound on other
> journeys.
>
> (Charles Dickens, *A Christmas Carol*)

Tomorrow's medicine is today's research. That is why the question
of how we allocate resources to research is at least as important as
the question of how we allocate resources to health care itself. But
this is not a question that you will find has been the focus of much
ethical discussion. Most discussion about the ethics of medical
research addresses the question of how research should be
regulated. Indeed, medical research is in many ways much more
strictly regulated than medical practice. From a perusal of the
innumerable guidelines on medical research you could be forgiven
for thinking that medical research, like smoking, must be bad for
your health; that in a liberal society, since it cannot be altogether
banned, strict regulation is needed to minimize the harm that it
can do.

The reason for this strict control lies in history. The appalling
experiments carried out by some Nazi doctors led, in 1946, to the

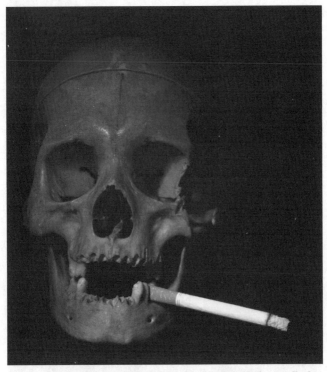

24. From reading the many guidelines you might think that medical research, like smoking, must be bad for your health.

first internationally agreed guidelines on medical research involving people – the Nuremberg Code. This code consisted of ten principles and these were incorporated by the medical profession into the Declaration of Helsinki, which was first published by the World Medical Association in 1964 and last updated in 2000. The Declaration of Helsinki has many offspring of varying legitimacy in the form of guidelines for medical research. These guidelines highlight four main issues: respect for the autonomy of the potential participants in research; the risk of harm; the value and quality of the research; and aspects of justice.

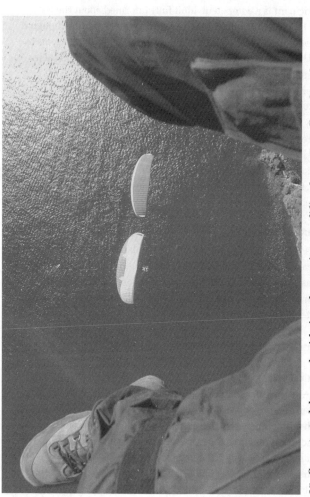

25. Competent adults can take risks in order to enjoy paragliding, but are not allowed to take comparable risks in order to help with medical research. Isn't this an infringement of our basic liberties?

The position taken on the risk of harm is rather interesting. Guidelines agree that research participants should not be put at more than 'minimal risk of harm'. This is the case even if the participant is a competent adult fully informed about the risks and benefits and who voluntarily agrees to take part. Although it is not entirely clear what is meant by minimal harm, it seems to be set at a level taken by somewhat risk-averse people in their normal lives. In other words the guidelines are highly paternalistic.

Why should risk of harm be more carefully controlled, and more restrictive, in the context of medical research, than it is in other areas of our lives? We do not prevent the sale or purchase of skis, motorbikes, or hang-gliders, although these expose purchasers to moderate risks. Why should the control of medical research be different?

Double standards

This is only one example where the regulation of medical research imposes standards that seem out of keeping with other areas of life. Another example is with regard to the amount of information provided to patients who are being asked to take part in a clinical trial.

Contrast these two situations:

Clinical case

Dr A sees patient B in the outpatient department. B is suffering from depression of a type likely to be helped with antidepressants. There are several slightly different antidepressants available. Dr A advises B to take a particular antidepressant (drug X) – the one with which he is most familiar and which is suitable for B. Dr A informs B about the likely benefits and the side effects of drug X. However, he says nothing about the other antidepressants that he could have prescribed instead.

Clinical trials

These are the standard method of assessing the value of a medical treatment. Suppose e.g. that the standard current treatment for disease D is drug X. A new drug, Y, has been developed. Preliminary studies suggest that Y may be an effective treatment for D, and possibly better than X. The best way to find out which drug is better is to give some patients with the disease drug X and others drug Y, and then see which group of patients does better. The group of patients receiving the new experimental drug (Y) is called the 'experimental' group. The group receiving the conventional treatment (X) is called the 'control' group. It is important that the two groups of patients (the experimental and control groups) are broadly similar. The trial results would be misleading if there were e.g. significantly more severely ill patients in one group than in the other group. The best way of ensuring that there are no significant differences between the groups is to use a random method ('tossing a coin') for allocating patients to each group, and to have a large number of patients in the trial. The best clinical trials are large randomized controlled trials (RCTs). When a treatment, such as a drug, is developed (treatment Y) for a condition where there is no current (conventional) treatment, the control group is given a 'placebo' – a dummy drug. Thus, if Y is a new drug that is taken as a tablet, the placebo would be a tablet that looks like the tablet containing Y but does not contain the active drug (Y). This is important because, for many conditions, patients can improve to some extent simply by believing that they are receiving active treatment. Doctors, furthermore, can be biased, when assessing a patient's improvement in health, by knowing whether the patient has been taking active treatment. It is therefore important that neither the patient nor the doctors know whether the patient is in the experimental or control groups.

Research case

A randomized controlled trial is under way to compare two antidepressants: drug X and drug Y. Although Dr A tends to prescribe drug X, on reflection he does not think that there is currently good evidence to prefer X to Y. It could be important to establish the relative effectiveness, and adverse effects, of each. Dr A therefore agrees to ask suitable patients whether they would be prepared to take part in the trial. Dr A sees B in the outpatient department. B is suffering from depression and would be a suitable candidate for the trial. In order to conform to the standards laid down by research ethics guidelines Dr A must obtain valid consent for B to enter the trial. He must inform B about the trial and its purpose. He must also inform B about both drugs X and Y and tell B that a random process will be used to choose which will be prescribed.

In the research case the guidelines and research ethics committees (also called institutional review boards) require Dr A to inform B about both drugs, and about the method of choosing which to prescribe. In the clinical case this standard of informing is not the norm. Is this difference justified? If it is, then the standards are simply different. If it is not then we are operating 'double standards' – i.e. standards that are different and where the difference is not justifiable. Double standards are an example of inconsistency. They tell us that at least one of the standards needs to be changed.

Medical research in the Third World

It is a third example of different standards on which I want to focus in this chapter. Under scrutiny here is not a comparison between research and ordinary life, nor between research and medical practice, but between research in rich countries and research in poor countries.

The Council for International Organizations of Medical Sciences laid down the following principle in its 1993 guidelines:

The ethical implications of research involving human subjects are identical in principle wherever the work is undertaken; they relate to respect for the dignity of each individual subject as well as to respect for communities, and protection of the rights and welfare of human subjects.

Marcia Angell, the former editor of the *New England Journal of Medicine*, wrote: 'Human subjects in any part of the world should be protected by an irreducible set of ethical standards.' Was this principle of equity breached by the following research studies? Angell thought that it was.

Preventing HIV transmission to infants in poor countries

The Human Immunovirus (HIV) causes the disease AIDS. A pregnant woman, infected with the HIV, may pass the infection on to her child. This is known as 'vertical transmission'. Treatment of a pregnant woman, infected with the HIV, with zidovudine (known as the ACTG 076 regimen) reduces the chance of vertical transmission. This regimen involves taking zidovudine by mouth (orally) during pregnancy, and being given it by injection into a vein during labour; and includes further doses to the newborn infant. This regimen is too expensive to be generally available in poor countries. A cheaper, but effective, regimen would potentially prevent a very large number of babies being infected with the HIV in poor countries. Without a cheaper regimen there is no available treatment in poor countries to prevent vertical transmission of HIV.

In 1997 the ACTG 076 regimen was the standard in the US because it was the only one that had been shown to be effective. It was thought possible that a cheaper regimen involving only oral zidovudine might be effective.

Two possible designs of trials to be carried out in poor countries are scientifically reasonable. The first is to compare the cheaper

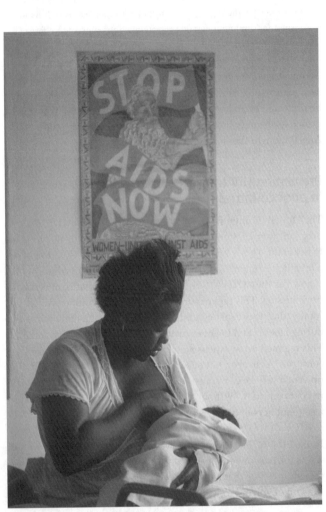

26. Will the 'ethical guidelines' that control international medical research slow down the development of effective treatments for those in poor countries?

regimen with a placebo. The second is to compare the cheaper regimen with the expensive regimen (ACTG 076). The first design is aimed at answering the question: is the cheap treatment better than nothing (placebo)? The second design is aimed at answering the question: is the cheap regimen as effective as the expensive regimen? In this case it was not realistic to introduce the expensive regimen as standard treatment into poor countries so the key question to be answered by the research was whether the cheaper regimen was better than nothing. This question can be answered more quickly, will involve fewer patients, and be cheaper using the first (placebo-controlled) design and it was this design that had been used in several studies, funded by rich countries, but conducted in poor countries.

It is generally accepted that the control group in a treatment trial should receive whatever is standard treatment (i.e. they should not be disadvantaged by the fact of taking part in the trial compared with people who are not in the trial). If you were taking part in a treatment trial in the UK or the US, a trial that was evaluating a new promising blood pressure drug, then you would be treated either with the new drug, or with what is current best treatment. You would not be given a placebo. That would be unethical because there is already known effective treatment.

Thus it would have been unethical in the sponsoring country (the US) to have carried out a placebo-controlled trial of the cheaper regimen because standard treatment in the US is the expensive (ACTG 076) regimen. On the principle of equity, therefore, many commentators thought that it was unethical to carry out a placebo-controlled study in the poor country: a double standard was operating. Furthermore the study was in breach of the Declaration of Helsinki which states that controls in treatment studies should receive the best current treatment.

But there are powerful arguments against this position. If the trial were conducted in a rich country it would be wrong for any patient

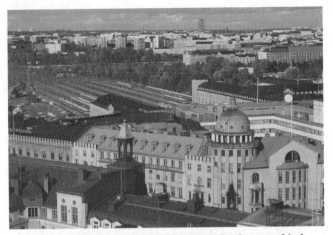

27. Helsinki: the Declaration of Helsinki provides the core ethical principles governing medical research across the world.

in the trial to receive placebo, since in normal clinical practice they would be receiving an active treatment. And this active treatment is known to be better than placebo. Now consider the case in a poor country. In normal clinical practice a patient would not receive any treatment. Indeed, many pregnant women infected with HIV would not receive any health care at all. The principle, stated in the Declaration of Helsinki, that those in the control arm should receive current best treatment is ambiguous. Does current best treatment mean best anywhere in the world, or best in the country where the research is being carried out? Those who believe that the placebo-controlled trial in the poor country was unethical think that the responsible ethics committee should not have allowed a trial using placebo control to be undertaken. But without the trial no one in the poor country would be receiving treatment to prevent vertical transmission. No one, therefore, receives worse treatment as a result of the placebo-controlled trial, and several people (those receiving the new treatment regimen) are likely to receive better treatment (although until the trial is carried out we don't know for certain that the new regimen is beneficial). And this is in marked contrast with the situation if a placebo-controlled trial were being carried out in a rich country, because in that case those given placebo would be worse off than patients not in the trial. In short, no one is harmed as a result of the placebo-controlled trial if it takes place in a poor country and some people stand to benefit.

The conclusion from this argument is that it would be better overall, for people in the poor country, that the placebo-controlled trial takes place. Those in the poor country also stand to benefit in the future from the trial as it may lead to the development of a treatment to prevent vertical transmission that is affordable for poor countries. If the trial were prevented from taking place, on the grounds that it is unethical because inequitable to people in poor countries, those in the poor country would be worse off. If equitable treatment means no treatment at all, give me inequitable treatment.

Against this it might be argued that, although the placebo-controlled trial is better than no trial, it would be better still to use the expensive regimen as control. But this would cost more. Who should pay? Perhaps those in rich countries should pay more to poor countries but it is not clear that this should be imposed on the sponsors of this research. Nor is it clear that the money is best spent on providing expensive HIV treatment for those who are allocated to the control arm of this trial. The extra money might be better spent in other ways – in ways, for example, that have greater beneficial effect on the health of those in poor countries.

In conclusion, the placebo study is not unethical – no one is harmed as a result of the study and some benefit. It would be worse for those in the poor country if the study did not take place. The principle stated in the Declaration of Helsinki and quoted above should be interpreted to mean that the control group should receive best treatment in the society in which the study takes place, not best treatment anywhere in the world. There is an ethical issue about the low level of health care available to those in poor countries – this is a major problem of justice. But this question needs to be tackled by governments and industry. This deep underlying and fundamental inequity should not be used to block research that, overall, benefits those in poor countries.

I have put forward two opposed positions.

1. That it is unethical to use a placebo control in a clinical trial carried out in a poor country when such a control would not be thought ethical had the research been carried out in a rich country. The ethics committee should not have allowed the trial described above to have taken place.
2. That the placebo control was not unethical, even if not ideal, and that it was right that the ethics committee allowed the trial to go ahead.

The first position seems to be on the side of the angels, making a bold claim of principle that those of us in rich countries should not treat people in poor countries any differently from ourselves. The second position uses the cold knife of rational argument to cut through our humane intuition and show that it is misguided. What should we do when rational argument contradicts humane intuition? The answer must be: re-examine both our intuitions and our arguments. Why does the first position seem to be on the side of the angels? Because we feel that it is treating those who are less privileged than ourselves as we would be treated. If we act according to the second view we have a niggling feeling that we are exploiting the poor. But the criticism of the first position seems valid: that by being precious about setting the same standards in poor countries that we would in rich countries we are making a decision (stopping the research) that will take away benefit from the very people towards whom we are wanting to be fair.

The clue to the way out of this impasse lies in the phrase 'exploiting the poor'. Someone can benefit from something but still be exploited. Consider coffee pickers in South America employed by an international company and paid low wages. Without such employment they may be even worse off. But if the company is making large profits, it is exploiting the pickers. The benefits should be fairly shared: that is what 'Fairtrade' is all about. Both of the opposed positions that we have been considering are too narrow.

The first position is right in highlighting the issue of equity, an issue closely related to exploitation. But it is wrong in blindly applying a principle (that controls should be given best treatment) that has been developed in a quite different context. The second position is right in showing that applying the principle is not in the best interests of those in poor countries, but it is wrong in considering only two possibilities. A much broader perspective is needed, and the starting point for that broader perspective is that the overarching ethical concern is the huge disparity in wealth and health care between rich and poor countries.

The implications of this perspective for international medical research include: (a) that the research must be conducted in ways that provide appropriate benefits to those in the poor country; and the benefits between rich and poor must be appropriately shared; (b) that a realistic view be taken as to what can be sustained in the poor country in order to properly evaluate how the benefits to poor countries can be maximized; (c) that the researchers have responsibilities not only to those in the poor countries who take part in the research but to the wider population. A public health perspective is therefore needed. A narrow focus on the best interests of the research participants only, without regard to the population, is excessively individualistic.

Henry Ford famously said: 'History is more or less bunk'. It has also been said, although I do not by whom: 'Those who are ignorant of history are condemned to repeat it'. The current international regulation of medical research grows, distorted by the long shadow of the Nazi past. This regulation is reactive, and obsessed with one main concern: to protect research participants from being abused. Important though this is there has been a failure to tackle the ethical implications of asking the constructive question: how can the good from medical research be maximized? Nowhere is this constructive approach more urgently needed than in research in poor countries.

Benatar and Singer write:

> There is thus a need to go beyond the reactive research ethics of the past. A new, proactive research ethics must be concerned with the greatest ethical challenge – the huge inequalities in global health.

Precisely so.

Chapter 9
Family medicine meets the House of Lords

Out of timber so crooked as that from which man is made nothing entirely straight can be built.

(Immanuel Kant)

Medical ethics deals, as we have seen, with some of the big issues of life, and death. It faces the extraordinary, both natural and man-made: conjoined twins, madness, assisted reproduction, cloning. Were you to base your understanding of medical ethics on the cases that hit the headlines you might think it a discipline concerned almost exclusively with the bizarre.

Doctors need to make judgements involving ethical values in the day-to-day practice of medicine, even in something as mundane as the treatment of raised blood pressure. For example, at what pressure should the patient be offered treatment? A population perspective might suggest that treatment of quite mild hypertension would prevent many people from suffering a stroke. For an individual the small reduction in absolute risk of stroke may not be worth the side effects of treatment. What factors should influence the choice of anti-hypertensive? How many of the possible side effects should the doctor reveal? Is there a danger that by mentioning some of the possible side effects, such as lassitude, the patient will be more likely to suffer them? Should the doctor accept the free dinner, with educational talk, from the manufacturer of one

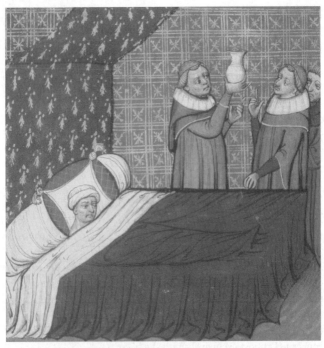

28. **Ethical issues arise in the practice of ordinary everyday medicine.**

of the principal anti-hypertensive drugs? Might this affect her prescribing decisions for the wrong reasons?

In this final chapter I want to look at two situations that most family doctors will have had to face. The ethical issues do not arise from any modern technology but from a problem only too familiar to health professionals: that families rarely enjoy the uncomplicated, easy, and unremittingly happy relationships that advertisements from the 1950s might lead you to expect.

The sixteenth-century essayist, Montaigne, a man who could write as comfortably about male impotence as on the education of children, had 57 maxims carved on the wooden beams of his study.

They included Terence's bold statement, which should perhaps be engraved on the stethoscopes of doctors: 'Nothing human is alien to me'. Difficult to achieve, of course, but a worthy aspiration for those whose jobs are aimed at helping people through difficult times. A tolerance of, perhaps even a fondness for, human frailty – Kant's crooked timber of humanity – is an important virtue in a health professional.

> The web of our life is of a mingled yarn, good and ill together; our virtues would be proud if our faults whipp'd them not, and our crimes would despair if they were not cherish'd by our virtues.
>
> (Shakespeare, *All's Well That Ends Well*, Act IV. Iii. 68–71)

What should the family doctor do when faced with the following situation?

Case: Dementia

Mr C is a 70-year-old man with dementia and long-standing lung disease (chronic obstructive pulmonary disease). He is cared for at home by his 72-year-old wife. He has frequent chest infections for which he receives antibiotics and he requires oxygen at home because of his lung disease. His most recent chest infection has not responded well to antibiotic tablets and his general condition is deteriorating. He is not eating and is drinking little. It is possible that, with hospital treatment, including intravenous antibiotics and physiotherapy, he may recover from this infection, although he is bound to develop a similar infection again in the near future. Admission to hospital in the past has caused him distress because he does not cope well with changing environments. His wife, however, says that she thinks that he should go to hospital so he can be given maximum treatment.

Imagine that you are the doctor and you think that Mr C's best interests would be served by his staying at home and being made comfortable. He is likely to die very soon at home; but he is likely to

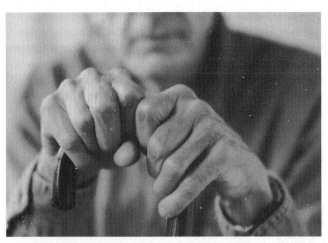

29. Home or hospital care? Who is to decide, and how?

die within a few months whatever happens. Because of his dementia his life is much less rich than the life that he used to lead. A few months of extra life in his state is just not worthwhile, particularly given the distress that hospital admission will cause him.

You think it is best for him to remain at home; his wife wants him in hospital. Where do you go from there?

There are common variations on this situation.

Variation 1

Mr C's wife agrees with you that the best thing to do would be for Mr C to remain at home, but their daughter, who lives close by, insists that he go into hospital to be given the best chance to recover from this episode of infection. Mrs C seems partly persuaded by her daughter, or perhaps a little bullied.

Variation 2

You, the doctor, think that if he goes into hospital he will recover and return to his usual level of health and that he may live for a year or so longer. You judge his life, although limited because of the dementia, to be nevertheless a happy one. This is partly because his wife looks after him so well. You think that it is in his best interests to go to hospital, but his wife says that she doesn't want him moved from home. She wants to nurse him, even if he will soon die. Perhaps that is what he would have wanted.

How should you think about the question of what is the right thing to do in these situations? In this book I have emphasized rational analysis. On such an approach a good starting place would be to identify some of the issues that might be important. For example, some of the issues that are raised by this case and its variations include the following.

1. Whether Mr C himself is able to form and express a view. This will depend principally on the degree of impairment from the dementia.
2. If Mr C is not now competent to form a view, is it possible to make some judgment about what he would have wanted in this situation?
3. What is in Mr C's best interests? If Mr C is himself competent to decide then his view of his best interests should normally prevail, but if Mr C is not competent to decide for himself the doctor will have to come to a view on what are Mr C's best interests. This may be a difficult issue. Is there a danger that the doctor will believe that because of the dementia Mr C's current life is not worth living and therefore it is better for him to be kept comfortable at home? Or is the danger the reverse: that a doctor feels the imperative to treat the infection and to keep Mr C alive. How can any person who is healthy judge what it is like to suffer dementia?
4. Should Mrs C's best interests be taken into account by the doctor or should he focus only on the patient's best interests?
5. Does Mrs C have some kind of right to decide what should happen to Mr C because she is the next of kin?
6. In the case of a disagreement within the family (e.g. a disagreement between Mrs C and her daughter) should the doctor give more

weight to the opinion of one person, e.g. Mrs C, and if so under what circumstances and for what reasons?

Such a list of issues is only the beginning of the analysis. Questions will then arise as to how to balance different aspects; but it makes perfect sense to start with such an analysis.

An alternative to this analytic approach is that of negotiation. Many clinicians would start, not with analysis, but with discussion. Such clinicians might begin by asking Mrs C why she thought that Mr C should go into hospital. What is important for these clinicians is understanding the needs, wishes, and perspectives of all those involved, and working towards an agreed decision that avoids conflicts: not always possible, of course, but with skill and patience it is often successful. In other words, this approach involves negotiation between the key people. It is an approach that most of us are familiar with in our everyday lives. It is how many families might decide what to do on a Sunday afternoon.

The distinction between using analysis and using negotiation in order to come to a decision is not absolute. Both require a mixture of analysis and of discussion. But they are at different ends of a spectrum. Negotiation brings in a perspective on medical ethics that I have not discussed elsewhere in this book. Most of this book, if I can caricature my own position, sees medical ethics as a question of working out the right action to take through reasoning. The reasoning process can be complex and there is no single method for carrying it out. Different problems require different tools. But this view sees medical ethics as essentially an individualistic enterprise: it is for individuals to decide what they believe is the right thing to do. The negotiation approach sees medical ethics – and indeed ethics in general – as essentially a process of interactions between people.

The ways in which health professionals should engage with

patients' families are even more complicated when the patient is not yet fully adult. I want now to consider another situation familiar to family doctors: the case of the 15-year-old pregnant girl.

Case: 15-year-old pregnant girl

A 15-year-old girl comes shyly to her primary care doctor, with a school friend for support. She thinks she is pregnant. Tests reveal that she is: about ten weeks pregnant. She wants an abortion. She is adamant that she does not want her parents to know.

The family doctor should talk to her, of course, although there is an immediate issue of whether the friend should or should not be present. With support and kindness the pregnant girl may come to agree to include her parents in the discussion. Even then the doctor may face difficult ethical issues, for example, the fraught issue of abortion itself. Suppose the doctor has a profound moral objection to abortion, but works in a country where in these circumstances it is legal. If both the girl and her parents want her to be referred to a gynaecologist for an abortion what should the doctor do? Try and persuade the family to change its mind, in which case how persuasive should he be? Or is his moral duty to inform only of the issues and let the family decide?

So, lurking behind this case are the complicated issues both of the morality of abortion, and of what doctors should do when faced with a conflict between professional duties and personal morality.

But neither of these issues is the one on which I want to focus. I want to look at the question of whether the doctor should ever refer the 15-year-old pregnant girl for an abortion without the parents' knowledge. Does the girl have a right to confidentiality? Do the parents have a right to know?

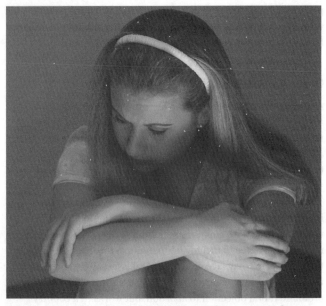

30. A 15-year-old is pregnant but doesn't want her parents to know. Should the doctor keep her confidence or tell her parents? (Posed by model.)

Thucydides' *History of the Peloponnesian Wars*, written in the 5th century BC is a treasure trove for those who love practical reasoning. The Athenian citizens expected carefully reasoned argument before waging war on their neighbours – how different from the sound-bite politics of modern democracies. Each side is given time to put its case without interruption. We can still enjoy this measured oral tradition of ethical reasoning in the legal judgements of our more senior courts.

Parental rights and medical consent, with respect to children under 16 years, was at the heart of a key English legal judgment: the Gillick case.

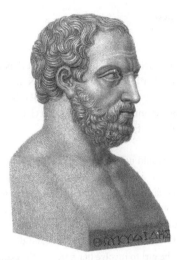

31a. Thucydides' bust.

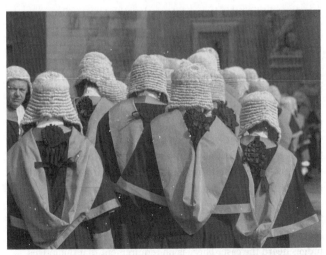

31b. The oral tradition of ethical reasoning is beautifully illustrated in Thucydides' *History*, written two and a half thousand years ago; and is still alive and well, and to be found in the House of Lords.

The Gillick case

The facts

In England, in the early 1980s the government department responsible for the National Health Service (NHS) – the Department of Health and Social Security (DHSS) – issued written advice for doctors about family planning services. This advice included two statements.

(a) That a doctor would not be acting unlawfully if he prescribed contraceptives for a girl under 16 years old, provided that he was acting in good faith to protect her against the harmful effects of sexual intercourse.

(b) That a doctor should normally only give contraception to a girl under 16 with the consent of the parents and that he should try to persuade the girl to involve her parents. Nevertheless, in exceptional cases a doctor could prescribe contraceptives without consulting the parents or obtaining their consent if in the doctor's clinical judgement it was desirable to prescribe contraceptives.

A private citizen, Mrs Victoria Gillick, sought assurance that none of her daughters would be given contraception without her knowledge and consent while they were under 16 years. The relevant NHS authority refused to give such assurance, saying that the issue was part of the clinical judgement for doctors. Mrs Gillick then brought legal action against the DHSS on the grounds that the advice to doctors was unlawful in allowing doctors to provide contraception to girls under 16 years without parental consent.

The case was eventually heard in England's highest court (equivalent to the US Supreme Court): the House of Lords. Five judges heard the case. There is no requirement that the judges agree. The final decision goes with the majority of judges. Each judge delivers his judgement, giving not only his decision but also the reasoning for it. Although the judges are answering the question of what is the correct legal position, and not the question: what is ethically right, the judgements are superb examples of ethical reasoning.

The judgements

Lord Brandon

Lord Brandon came down on the side of Mrs Gillick. Indeed he went further. He concluded that to give contraception to a girl under 16 years, even with the knowledge and consent of the parent(s), was unlawful. His argument, in a nutshell, was as follows:

1. It is a legal fact (because of a statute in English law) that a man who has sexual intercourse with a girl under 16 years, even with the consent of the girl, commits a criminal act.
2. It is also a criminal act to encourage or facilitate a criminal act.
3. Giving a girl contraception or advice about contraception involves encouraging the girl to have sexual intercourse with a man. It amounts to encouraging a criminal act.
4. Some might argue that some girls will have intercourse whether or not they are given contraception, and in such a case the giving of contraception is not encouraging the girl to have intercourse. But this is mistaken for two reasons. First, the fact that the girl is seeking contraception shows that she is aware of, and potentially discouraged from intercourse by, the risk of unwanted pregnancy. Thus, Brandon argues, she and her partner are more likely to 'indulge their desire' if contraception is given. Second, if the law allows a girl under 16 years to get contraception if she convinces her parents and doctor that she will have (unlawful) intercourse anyway, then the girl can essentially blackmail or threaten her parents and doctor to get her own way. Brandon writes: 'The only answer which the law should give to such a threat is, "Wait till you are 16"'.

Lord Templeman

Lord Templeman also supported Gillick, although he took a different position from Lord Brandon. He did not consider it necessarily illegal for a girl less than 16 years to be given contraception if both the doctor and the parent(s) agree that this is in her best interests. He believed that there might be situations where a girl cannot be deterred from illegal sexual intercourse and that providing contraception for the purpose of avoiding an unwanted pregnancy was not encouraging or aiding the illegal act.

But he did not believe that doctors should have the clinical discretion to provide contraception in this situation without the parents' consent. He based this position on four arguments.

1.   That a girl under 16 years is not competent to give consent to contraception. He wrote: 'I doubt whether a girl under the age of 16 is capable of a balanced judgment to embark on . . . sexual intercourse.' He gave legal reasons for this position. He argued that, since it is illegal for a man to have sexual intercourse with a girl under 16 years old even with that girl's consent the law must consider such consent as invalid.

2.   That the doctor can never be in a position to properly judge whether or not it is in the best interests of the girl to be given contraception without information from the parents.

3.   One of the duties of parents is to protect their children from illegal intercourse through persuasion, the exercise of parental power, or through influencing the relevant man. If the doctor gives contraception without informing the parents then he is interfering with the parents' ability to carry out their duty.

4.   That parents have rights to know by virtue of being parents.

. . . the parent who knows most about the girl and ought to have the most influence with the girl is entitled to exercise parental rights of control, supervision, guidance and advice in order that the girl may, if possible, avoid sexual intercourse until she is older.

For a doctor to keep the girl's confidence 'would constitute an unlawful interference with the rights of the parent' to make that decision and with 'the right of the parent to influence the conduct of the girl by the exercise of parental power of control, guidance, and advice'.

'There are many things which a girl under 16 needs to practice', he writes, 'but sex is not one of them'. I suppose he was thinking of piano practice.

Two judges in favour of Gillick. Three judges to go.

Lord Fraser

Lord Fraser disagreed with both the previous judges and with Gillick and came down in favour of the DHSS. He distinguishes three strands of argument.

1. Whether a girl under the age of 16 has the legal capacity to give valid consent to contraceptive advice and treatment.
2. Whether the giving of such advice and treatment to a girl under 16 without her parents' consent infringes the parents' rights.
3. Whether a doctor who gives such advice or treatment to a girl under 16 without her parents' consent incurs criminal liability.

He considers these in order. On the question of legal capacity to give valid consent Lord Fraser considers various pieces of legislation and concludes that none gives legal grounds for necessarily considering someone under 16 as lacking capacity to consent to medical treatment, including contraceptive treatment. With regard to the argument made by Lord Templeman he draws the opposite conclusion. He argues that 'a girl under 16 can give sufficiently effective consent to sexual intercourse to lead to the legal result that the man involved does not commit the crime of rape' (although he still commits a lesser crime).

Lord Fraser argues that the legal basis for parental rights to control a child exist

> for the benefit of the child and they are justified only in so far as they enable the parent to perform his duties towards the child. . . . the degree of parental control actually exercised over a particular child does in practice vary considerably according to his understanding and intelligence and it would, in my opinion, be unrealistic for the courts not to recognise these facts. Social customs change, and the law ought to, and does in fact, have regard to such changes when they are of major importance.

After considering various previous judgements Lord Fraser goes on to write:

> Once the rule of parents' absolute authority over minor children is abandoned, the solution to the problem in this appeal can no longer be found by referring to rigid parental rights at any particular age. The solution depends on a judgment of what is best for the welfare of the particular child. Nobody doubts, certainly I do not doubt, that in the overwhelming majority of cases the best judges of a child's welfare are his or her parents. Nor do I doubt that any important medical treatment of a child under 16 would normally only be carried out with the parents' approval. But . . . Mrs Gillick . . . has to justify the absolute right of veto in a parent. But there may be circumstances in which a doctor is a better judge of the medical advice and treatment which will conduce to a girl's welfare than her parents. It is notorious that children of both sexes are often reluctant to confide in their parents about sexual matters . . . There may well be . . . cases where the doctor feels that . . . there is no realistic prospect of her [the girl under 16] abstaining from intercourse. If that is right it points strongly to the desirability of the doctor being entitled in some cases, in the girl's best interest, to give her contraceptive advice and treatment if necessary without the consent or even the knowledge of her parents.

He dismisses the view held by Lord Brandon that a doctor would be committing a criminal offence under the Sexual Offences Act 1956 by aiding and abetting the commission of unlawful sexual intercourse in giving contraception, or contraceptive advice, to girls under 16.

> It would depend on the doctor's intentions; this appeal is concerned with doctors who honestly intend to act in the best interests of the girl, and I think it is unlikely that a doctor who gives contraceptive advice or treatment with that intention would commit an offence . . .

Lord Scarman

Lord Scarman considers the issue of the capacity of children under 16 years in more detail than Lord Fraser:

> I would hold that as a matter of law the parental right to determine whether or not their minor child below the age of 16 will have medical treatment terminates if and when the child achieves a sufficient understanding and intelligence to enable him or her to understand fully what is proposed.

He concludes that the guidance from the DHSS can be followed without involving the doctor in any infringement of parental right.

Scarman is in agreement with Fraser. Two all with one to go.

Lord Bridge

Lord Bridge raises an issue that is not covered directly in any of the other judgements. He is concerned with the role of legal judgement in cases where there are ethical and social issues, as in the case being examined. He writes:

> if a government department . . . promulgates . . . advice which is erroneous in law, then the court . . . has jurisdiction to correct the error of law . . . In cases where any proposition of law . . . is interwoven with questions of social and ethical controversy, the

court should, in my opinion, exercise its jurisdiction with the utmost restraint, confine itself to deciding whether the proposition of law is erroneous and avoid . . . expressing ex cathedra opinions in areas of social and ethical controversy in which it has no claim to speak with authority . . .

Having given this warning he takes issue with Lord Brandon and agrees with Lords Fraser and Scarman.

The DHSS wins, Gillick loses: three Lords to two.

Notes and references

Chapter 1

Ice-cream stall owner, in M. Pryce *Aberystwyth Mon Amour*
(Bloomsbury: London, 2001)

See W. H. Auden's poem: Musée des Beaux Arts. Faber and Faber,
1979

Isaiah Berlin, *The Hedgehog and the Fox* (Weidenfeld & Nicolson,
1953)

As written by Zadie Smith in the *Guardian* (London) review
(1 Nov. 2003), p. 6

Chapter 2

Thucydides, *History of the Peloponnesian War*, tr. R. Warner,
(Penguin: London, 1954)

Warburton N, *Thinking from A to Z*, 2nd edn. (Routledge, 1996)

Colin Spencer, *Heretic's Feast: A History of Vegetarianism* (University
Press of New England, 1996)

J. Rachels, 'Active and Passive Euthanasia', *New England Journal of
Medicine*, 292 (1975), 78–80; reprinted in P. Singer (ed.), *Applied
Ethics* (Oxford University Press, 1986) – for the cases of Smith and
Jones

J. Glover, *Causing Death and Saving Lives* (Penguin, 1977), p. 93 – for
the cases of Robinson and Davies (originally from an article by P. Foot)

For a detailed account of the Cox case, see I. Kennedy and A. Grubb,
Medical Law, 3rd edn. (Butterworths, 2000)

Chapter 3

J. S. Mill on Bentham in *London and Westminster Review*, 1838; reprinted in *Dissertations and Discussions I*, 1859

Tony Bullimore's account of his rescue is given in *Saved* (Time Warner Books, 1997). Calculating the cost of the rescue is not at all straightforward, as Bullimore himself discusses (p. 293). One could put a price on all the person-hours, the airplane, and ship usage. This would probably come to several million pounds. Alternatively you might argue that all the personnel would have been paid anyway – so the only extra cost was the wear and tear on the planes and ships. Or you could say that the rescue was useful training and cost-free. In many situations the cost estimation of health care interventions are similarly open to enormous variation depending on what is included in the calculation.

Chapter 4

Laurence Sterne, *The Life and Opinions of Tristram Shandy, Gentleman* (1760; Everyman Library), chs. 2 and 1

The Human Fertilisation and Embryology Act, section 13(5)

I. Kennedy and A. Grubb, *Medical Law* (3rd edn. Butterworths, 2000), pp. 1272–3

Montesquieu said that 'Men should be mourned at their birth, and not at their death' (Il faut pleurer les hommes a leur naissance, et non pas a leur mort)

D. Parfit, *Reasons and Persons* (Oxford University Press, 1984), ch. 16

Chapter 5

J. L. Borges, 'The Art of Verbal Abuse', tr. S. J. Levine, *The Total Library* ed. by E. Weinberger (Viking: London and New York, 1999)

J. Rawls, *A Theory of Justice* (Oxford University Press, 1972)

Flew, *An Introduction to Western Philosophy* (Thames and Hudson, 1989)

R. Gillon, *Philosophical Medical Ethics* (Wiley & Son, 1986)

G. Priest, *Logic: A Very Short Introduction* (Oxford University Press, 2000)

Chapter 6

N. Gogol 'Diary of a Madman', 1835 tr. C. English *Plays and Petersburg Tales* (Oxford University Press, 1995)

The discussion on protecting society from dangerous people owes a great deal to Harriet Mather who developed many of these ideas in the course of her studies as a medical student.

L. Reznek, *The Nature of Disease* (Routledge & Kegan Paul, 1987)

B v Croydon District Health Authority (1994) 22 BMLR 13

Chapter 7

M. Montaigne, 'On the Resemblance of Children to their Fathers', *The Complete Essays* tr. M. A. Screech (Allen Lane, The Penguin Press, 1991)

M. Parker and A. Lucassen, *Lancet*, 357 (2001), 1033–5, for the cases concerning paternity

President's Commission on the Ethical Issues of Genetic Testing *Am Med News* 26 (1983) p. 25

Institute of Medicine, Committee on Assessing Genetic Risks, Assessing Genetic Risks (National Academy Press, 1994), p. 276

D. C. Wertz, J. C. Fletcher, and J. J. Mulvihill, 'Medical Geneticists Confront Ethical Dilemmas: Cross-Cultural Comparisons among 18 Nations', *American Journal of Human Genetics*, 46 (1990), 1200–13

General Medical Council 2000 Confidentiality: Protecting and Providing Information www.gmc-uk.org

M. Parker and A. Lucassen, 'Genetic Information: A Joint Account?', *BMJ* (in press)

Chapter 8

C. Dickens *A Christmas Carol*, 1843

T. Hope and J. McMillan, 'Challenge Studies of Human Volunteers: Ethical Issues', *Journal of Medical Ethics 30* (2004) p. 110–116, for standard of 'minimal harm'

I. Chalmers and R. I. Lindley, 'Double Standards on Informed Consent to Treatment', in L. Doyal and J. S. Tobias (eds.), *Informed Consent in Medical Research* (BMJ Books, 2001), pp. 266–76

Council for International Organizations of Medical Sciences (CIOMS) in collaboration with the World Health Organization (WHO) Geneva, *International Ethical Guidelines for Biomedical Research Involving Human Subjects* (1993)

The 1993 guidelines were superseded by revised guidelines in 2002 (www.cioms.ch/frame_guidelines_nov_2002.htm). The revision was, in part, in response to the controversy following the study considered in the second part of this chapter. The members of the group who wrote the revised guidelines were unable to agree over the issues discussed. It is interesting to read the varying opinions (see website above)

M. Angell, 'Ethical Imperialism? Ethics in International Collaborative Clinical Research', *New England Journal of Medicine*, 319 (1988), 1081–3

P. Lurie and S. M. Wolf, 'Unethical Trials of Interventions to Reduce Perinatal Transmission of the Human Immunodeficiency Virus in Developing Countries', *New England Journal of Medicine*, 337 (1997), 853–6

A good way of following the debate on trials in poor countries is to start with the following article that is available on the BMJ website through searching the archive (http://bmj.bmjjournals.com/) Many of the key articles are available free online and can be accessed from the reference list at the end of the following article: Solomon R. Benatar and Peter A. Singer, 'A New Look at International Research Ethics', *BMJ* 321 (Sept. 2000), 824–6.

For an excellent discussion of exploitation see A. Wertheimer, *Exploitation* (Princeton University Press, 1996).

Chapter 9

I. Kant, 'Idee zu einer allgemeinen Geschichte in weltbürgerlicher Absicht', tr. I. Berlin, in *The Crooked Timber of Humanity* (Fontana Press, 1991)

Further reading

I hope that this 'taster' of medical ethics has whetted your appetite for the subject. I have provided further reading for specific topics in each chapter below. First I will recommend more general books and journals.

The methods of medical ethics are of course those of ethics more generally; it is the subject matter that is specific. Having said that, medical ethics is one area of practical ethics that has been particularly innovative in its methodologies. A developing area is the use of empirical methods in medical ethics: collecting data about the real world using, principally, methods borrowed from the social sciences. Empirical research and philosophical analysis can be closely integrated to enrich both. A good book that discusses the use of different methods is: J. Sugarman and D. Sulmasy (eds.), *Methods in Medical Ethics* (Georgetown University Press, 2001).

If you want to delve into general ethical theories and approaches then a good collection of essays on a wide variety of ethical theories is: P. Singer, *A Companion to Ethics* (Blackwell Reference, 1991).

W. Kymlica, *Contemporary Political Philosophy: An Introduction* (Oxford University Press, 1990) summarizes six types of political philosophy: utilitarianism; liberal equality; libertarianism; marxism; communitarianism; and feminism. Although the summaries are short, the level of analysis is philosophically sophisticated.

There are several good encyclopedias of ethics that provide good introductions to a particular topic with good reference lists. Examples are:

R. F. Chadwick (ed.), *Encyclopedia of Applied Ethics*, 4 vols. (Academic Press, 1998)

L. C. Becker (ed.), *Encyclopedia of Ethics* (Garland, 1992)

P. Edwards (ed.), *The Encyclopedia of Philosophy* (Macmillan and Free Press, 1972)

Two contrasting types of ethical theory are worth exploring: duty-based theories and utilitarianism. Three chapters in Singer (ed.), *A Companion to Ethics* (see above), provide clear and fairly detailed accounts of various duty-based approaches to ethics: 'Kantian Ethics' by Onora O'Neill (pp. 175–85), 'Contemporary Deontology' by Nancy Davis (pp. 205–18), 'An Ethic of Prima Facie Duties' by Jonathan Dancy (pp. 219–29). For a short but rigorous account of Kant's moral theory see R. Walker, *Kant and the Moral Law* (Phoenix Orion Publishing Group, 1998), pp. 39–42. The most accessible of Kant's own writings on ethics is: I. Kant, *Groundwork of the Metaphysics of Morals*, tr. and ed. M. Gregor (Cambridge University Press, 1998).

Key essays by the founders of utilitarianism, Jeremy Bentham and John Stuart Mill, including Mill's classic essay, are found in: *Utilitarianism and Other Essays: J.S. Mill and J. Bentham*, ed. A Ryan (Penguin, 1987). A clear and wide-ranging book that provides a useful and up-to-date analysis of utilitarianism is: R. Crisp, *Mill on Utilitarianism* (Routledge, 1997). A short introduction to utilitarianism and its philosophical problems is given in: J. J. C. Smart and B. Williams, *Utilitarianism for and against* (Cambridge University Press, 1973).

Many modern medical ethicists, and also health care professionals, find the approach of 'virtue ethics' useful and interesting. This approach derives from Aristotle and focuses on the character of the people who are faced with the difficult ethical issues. A book that collects together several articles using a virtue ethics approach, some of which are in the field of medical ethics, is: R. Crisp and M. Slote (eds.), *Virtue Ethics* (Oxford Readings in Philosophy; Oxford University Press, 1997). The editors' introduction gives a good analysis of virtue ethics.

A short introduction to medical ethics that takes a quite different approach from this book is: R. Gillon, *Philosophical Medical Ethics* (Wiley & Son, 1996). Gillon's book structures the analysis of medical ethics around the 'four principles' (see p. 65–66) and relates these to clinical practice. For a much larger textbook of medical ethics that pioneered this four-principle approach see: T. L. Beauchamp and J. F. Childress, *Principles of Biomedical Ethics*, 5th edn. (Oxford University Press, 2001), which is the world's best-selling medical ethics textbook.

Other good general books in medical ethics are:

J. Glover, *Causing Death and Saving Lives* (Penguin, 1977): although this is about end of life issues it is a good introduction to philosophical thinking applied to the medical setting

J. Harris, *The Value of Life* (Routledge & Kegan Paul, 1985)

P. Singer, *Practical Ethics*, 2nd edn. (Cambridge University Press, 1993): a racy and readable examination of some of the philosophical issues underpinning medical ethics

M. Parker and D. Dickenson, *The Cambridge Medical Ethics Workbook* (Cambridge University Press, 2001): this provides many cases taken from health care across several European countries, together with analysis of the cases – a combination of textbook and case book

A. Campbell, M. Charlesworth, Grant Gillett and Gareth Jones, *Medical Ethics* (Oxford University Press, 1997): accessible and relatively small textbook written by a team of philosophers and doctors

Medical Ethics Today: The BMA's Handbook of Ethics and Law (British Medical Association, 2004): more medical in its orientation than most textbooks of medical ethics

K. Boyd, R. Higgs, and A. Pinching, *The New Dictionary of Medical Ethics* (BMJ Books, 1997): an alphabetical list of terms and concepts in medical ethics

Together with colleagues, I have written a textbook in medical ethics and law aimed primarily at medical students and doctors: T. Hope, J. Savulescu, and J. Hendrick, *Medical Ethics and Law: The Core Curriculum* (Churchill Livingstone, 2003).

If you want to read some classic papers in medical ethics, the following are useful collections.

J. D. Arras and Bonnie Steinbock, *Ethical Issues in Modern Medicine*, 6th edn. (McGraw-Hill, 2002)

T. Beauchamp and L. Walters (eds.), *Contemporary Issues in Bioethics*, 5th edn. (Wadsworth Publishing Co., 1999)

M. Freeman (ed.), *Ethics and Medical Decision-Making* (Ashgate, 2001)

H. Kuhse and P. Singer (eds.), *Bioethics: An Anthology* (Blackwell Publishers, 1999)

The following are case books in medical ethics: G. E. Pence, *Classic Cases in Medical Ethics*, 2nd edn. (McGraw-Hill, 1994); G. E. Pence, *Classic Works in Medical Ethics: Core Philosophical Readings* (McGraw-Hill, 1998).

The academic world shares ideas through journals as much as through books, or discussion. Many of the articles, although by no means all, are readily accessible to the interested lay reader. The *Journal of Medical Ethics* aims at health professionals as much as at philosophers, and publishes clinical case studies, relevant social science as well as ethical argument. It also has a good website (see below). *Hastings Center Report* covers a wide range with social science and policy-oriented articles as well as more pure medical ethics.

Two other major international journals in medical ethics with a mainly philosophical perspective are: *Bioethics* and the *Kennedy Institute of Ethics Journal*. The *Bulletin of Medical Ethics* provides up-to-date news items and has short articles including briefing articles about, for example, media stories or parliamentary debates. The *Journal of Applied Philosophy* covers applied philosophy generally. This includes such areas as environmental ethics, criminology, business ethics, as well as topics in medical ethics.

There are of course innumerable websites of relevance to medical ethics. Here are three that also offer good gateways to further sites:

http://jme.bmjjournals.com/ This leads to the *Journal of Medical Ethics* website

http://www.ethox.org.uk/ The website for the Ethox Centre – the Medical Ethics Centre in Oxford where I work

http://bioethics.georgetown.edu/ The website of the Kennedy Institute that has the largest medical ethics library in the world. This is a good portal for databases in medical ethics

Chapter 2

If you want to pursue some of the philosophical issues raised in this chapter such as the acts-omissions distinction, or if you want to think about a broader range of problems around the end of life then an excellent, readable and philosophically sophisticated discussion is given by J. Glover, *Causing Death and Saving Lives* (Penguin, 1977). Ronald Dworkin, in his book *Life's Dominion: An Argument about Abortion, Euthanasia, and Individual Freedom* (Vintage Books, 1993), links end of life issues, including abortion, to individual freedom, as its subtitle suggests. This is not a comprehensive account of the issues but the application of a set of related perspectives to end of life issues. A useful book that covers a wide range of issues in medicine at the end of life is: D. W. Brock, *Life and Death: Philosophical Essays in Biomedical Ethics* (Cambridge University Press, 1993).

If you want to read more about euthanasia and physician assisted suicide then the following three books are a good way in to the literature:

M. Battin, R. Rhodes, and A. Silvers (eds.), *Physician Assisted Suicide: Expanding the Debate* (Routledge, 1998)

G. Dworkin, R. G. Frey, and Sissela Bok, *Euthanasia and Physician-Assisted Suicide: For and Against* (Cambridge University Press, 1998)

J. Keown, *Euthanasia Examined* (Cambridge University Press, 1995)

Chapter 3

The argument against the 'rule of rescue' given in this chapter is based on: T. Hope, 'Rationing and Life-Saving Treatment: Should Identifiable Patients have Higher Priority?', *Journal of Medical Ethics*, 27/3 (2001), 179–85.

For a good collection of both practical and theoretical papers covering a wide range of contemporary issues in health care rationing see: A. Coulter and C. Ham (eds.), *The Global Challenge of Health Care Rationing* (Open University Press, 2000); and M. Battin, R. Rhodes, and A. Silvers (eds.), *Medicine and Social Justice* (Oxford University Press, 2002), which provides an up-to-date collection with perspectives from both sides of the Atlantic.

Cost-effectiveness analysis is a technique developed by health economists for trying to get a handle on comparing different types of treatment (or other health care intervention). The method aims at estimating the cost for a standardized unit of health gain. The most commonly used standardized unit is the 'Quality Adjusted Life Year' or QALY. A book that provides an up-to-date European perspective on QALYs in practice is: A. Edgar, S. Salek, D. Shickle, and D. Cohen, *The Ethical QALY: Ethical Issues in Healthcare Resource Allocations* (Euromed Communications, 1998). This book covers the measurement of QALYs, the ethical and technical difficulties with them, and contains a number of short summaries of health care rationing in various European countries, including some from the former Eastern Europe.

A detailed and quite technical book on the various kinds of cost-effectiveness which discusses both the ethical and economic aspects is: M. R. Gold, J. E. Siegel, L. B. Russell, and M. C. Weinstein (eds.), *Cost-Effectiveness in Health and Medicine* (Oxford University Press, 1996).

The *Journal of Medical Ethics* published an interesting and lively debate about the ethical strengths and weaknesses of the cost-effectiveness approach to rationing. J. Harris argued against QALY theory: 'QALYfying the Value of Human Life', *Journal of Medical Ethics*, 13 (1987), 117–23. P. Singer, J. McKie, H. Kuhse, and J. Richardson reply to Harris: 'Double Jeopardy and the Use of QALYs in Health Care Allocation', *Journal of Medical Ethics*, 21 (1995), 144–50. Harris defended his original position: 'Double Jeopardy and the Veil of Ignorance – a Reply', *Journal of Medical Ethics*, 21 (1995), 151–7. The debate is summarized by T. Hope: 'QALYs, Lotteries and Veils: The Story so Far', *Journal of Medical Ethics*, 22 (1996), 195–6. The debate then continued in three adjacent articles in the same volume:

J. McKie, H. Kuhse, J. Richardson, and P. Singer, 'Double Jeopardy, the Equal Value of Lives and the Veil of Ignorance: A Rejoinder to Harris', pp. 204–8

J. Harris, 'Would Aristotle have Played Russian Roulette?', pp. 209–15

J. McKie, H. Kuhse, J. Richardson, and P. Singer, 'Another Peep behind the Veil', *Journal of Medical Ethics*, pp. 216–21

Chapter 4

The first major exploration of the non-identity problem from a philosophical angle is in: D. Parfit, *Reasons and Persons* (Oxford University Press, 1984), ch. 16. A more extended analysis of the implications of the non-identity problem for doctors, with references to some of the more recent articles is given in: T. Hope and J. McMillan (2004) [in preparation].

An early and lively discussion of issues raised by the possibility of selecting the characteristics of our children is given in: J. Glover, *What*

Sort of People Should There Be? (Pelican, 1984). For more general coverage of ethical issues around assisting reproduction see: J. Harris and Soren Holm (eds.), *The Future of Human Reproduction: Ethics, Choice and Regulation* (Oxford University Press, 1998). This is a collection of essays. The introduction by Harris provides a useful overview of ethical issues in assisted reproduction. J. Robertson, *Children of Choice: Freedom and the New Reproductive Technologies* (Princeton University Press, 1994), provides an examination of a wide range of issues associated with assisted reproduction and the new genetics with extensive coverage of the associated literature.

The most obvious area of reproductive medicine that raises important ethical concerns is that of abortion. A brief overview of some of the main positions on abortion is given in: T. Hope, J. Savulescu, and J. Hendrick, *Medical Ethics and Law: The Core Curriculum* (Churchill-Livingstone, 2003), ch. 9. More detailed, but readable discussions are in: J. Glover, *Causing Death and Saving Lives* (Penguin, 1977) and R. Dworkin, *Life's Dominion: An Argument about Abortion, Euthanasia, and Individual Freedom* (Vintage Books, 1993). Two articles that provide perspectives on the morality of abortion that get away from the focus on the moral status of the embryo are: J. J. Thomson, 'A Defence of Abortion', *Philosophy and Public Affairs* (Princeton University Press, 1971), reprinted in P. Singer (ed.), *Applied Ethics* (Oxford University Press, 1986); R. Hursthouse, 'Virtue Theory and Abortion', *Philosophy and Public Affairs*. 20 (1991), 223–46, reprinted in R. Crisp and M. Slote (eds.), *Virtue Ethics* (Oxford University Press, 1997), pp. 217–38.

Chapter 5

Anne Thomson, *Critical Reasoning in Ethics* (Routledge, 1999), provides a clear and thorough examination of thinking about ethics with many examples. A useful source book of types of fallacy and of valid reasoning in a simple dictionary style is N. Warburton, *Thinking from A to Z* (Routledge, 1996). For an entertaining introduction to formal logic, see G. Priest, *Logic: A Very Short Introduction* (Oxford University Press,

2000). This book has a good account of the sorites paradox and the slippery slope argument, but, despite its brevity and accessibility, this sister book gets into some pretty technical stuff.

For a lively, but far from superficial, introduction to ethics, and ethical theory, see: S. Blackburn, *Ethics: A Very Short Introduction* (Oxford University Press, 2001). And if you want to take a further step back – from ethics to philosophy more generally – see: E. Craig, *Philosophy: A Very Short Introduction* (Oxford University Press, 2002). An excellent history of ethics, that is also an excellent introduction to the subject, is A. MacIntyre, *A Short History of Ethics* (Routledge Classics; Routledge, 2002).

The critical philosophical tradition – the tradition of argument – began in ancient Greece around the 6th century BC. An excellent introduction to Greek philosophy is: J. Annas, *Ancient Philosophy: A Very Short Introduction* (Oxford University Press, 2000). And why not dip into Plato himself, and meet Socrates as both questioner and orator. An engaging place to start is with the Plato dialogues that are sometimes brought together as the 'Trial and Death of Socrates': *Euthyphro*, *Apology* (an account of Socrates' trial, and one of the dramatic masterpieces), *Crito*, and *Phaedo* (which ends with Socrates' last words as the paralysing effect of hemlock creeps up his body). All four are available (together with a fifth dialogue) in Plato, *Five Dialogues: Euthyphro, Apology, Crito, Meno, and Phaedo*, tr. G. M. A. Grube (Hackett Publishing Co., 2002). The *Apology* and *Phaedo* are available as an audiobook from Naxos.

Chapter 6

The 'anti-psychiatry' movement of the 1960s produced some trenchant and well-written critiques of the whole idea of mental illness and the coercive ways in which society treats the mentally ill. Two of the most influential such books were: R. D. Laing, *The Divided Self* (Penguin Books, 1990; 1st publ. 1960), and T. Szasz, *The Myth of Mental Illness*, rev. edn. (Harper Collins, 1984; 1st publ. 1960). An excellent edited collection covering a wide range of areas of ethics and mental illness is:

R. Bloch, P. Chodoff, and S. A. Green, *Psychiatric Ethics*, 3rd edn. (Oxford University Press, 1999).

It is in the field of mental illness that philosophical issues about the concept of disease and classification have been most discussed. Two useful overviews of some key positions and arguments are found in C. Boorse, 'A Rebuttal on Health', in J. F. Humber and R. F. Almeder (eds.), *Defining Disease* (Humana Press, 1997), pp. 7–8, and K. W. M. Fulford, 'Analytic Philosophy, Brain Science, and the Concept of Disorder', in Bloch *et al.*, *Psychiatric Ethics*.

A good starting point for the literature on the abuse of psychiatry for political purposes is: P. Chodoff, 'Misuse and Abuse of Psychiatry: An Overview', in Bloch *et al.*, *Psychiatric Ethics*.

Although not discussed in this chapter, there are many ethical issues that arise from the practice of psychotherapy. These are discussed in some detail in J. Holmes and R. Lindley, *The Values of Psychotherapy* (Oxford University Press, 1991).

Chapter 7

The ethical issues that arise from modern genetics are the current growth industries of medical ethics. For an extensive list of further reading see: T. Hope, J. Savulescu, and J. Hendrick, *Medical Ethics and Law: The Core Curriculum* (Churchill-Livingstone, 2003), pp. 112–13.

British Medical Association, *Human Genetics: Choice and Responsibility* (Oxford University Press, 1998), gives the British Medical Association's position on ethics and genetics. An excellent book on ethics and the new genetics which thoroughly covers the literature is A. Buchanan, D. W. Brock, N. Daniels, and D. Wikler, *From Chance to Choice: Genetics and Justice* (Cambridge University Press, 2000). J. Harris, *Clones, Genes and Immortality* (Oxford University Press, 1998) is written in Harris's characteristically vigorous style.

Few can resist the lure of taking up a strong position on the ethics of human cloning. Perhaps not the stuff of ordinary clinical practice, but it is certainly good for discussion over a pint of beer. For a 'what is all the fuss about' approach read: J. Harris, '"Goodbye Dolly?" The Ethics of Human Cloning', *Journal of Medical Ethics*, 23 (1997), 353–60. For a collection of essays on cloning from a variety of perspectives: M. C. Nussbaum and C. R. Sunstein (eds.), *Clones and Clones: Facts and Fantasies about Human Cloning* (W. W. Norton & Co., 1998). For an overview of the history and facts as well as some of the philosophical issues see: A. J. Klotzko, *A Clone of your own?: The Science and Ethics of Cloning* (Oxford University Press, 2004).

For a good history of eugenics see: D. J. Kevles, *In the Name of Eugenics: Genetics and the Uses of Human Heredity* (Harvard University Press, 1995). A good overview and analysis of eugenics is provided in D. Wikler, 'Can we Learn from Eugenics?', *Journal of Medical Ethics*, 25/2 (1999), 183–94.

Prenatal diagnosis of genetic conditions that cause disability, followed by termination of pregnancy, has been the object of considerable criticism on the grounds not that termination is wrong *per se* but because this discriminates against the disabled. For a collection of papers on this issue, see: E. Parens and A. Asch (eds.), *Prenatal Testing and Disability Rights* (Georgetown University Press, 2000).

The time may not be far off when genetic methods can be used, not to prevent disease or disability, but to enhance humans – for example to increase intelligence. Most of us believe it is right to enhance children's intellectual abilities through good education. Is it right to enhance children's intelligence through gene therapy? If you want to read about this issue, try N. Holtug, 'Does Justice Require Genetic Enhancements?', *Journal of Medical Ethics*, 25/2 (1999), 137–43 and J. Savulescu, 'In defence of selection for non-disease genes.', *American Journal of Bioethics* 175 (2001) p. 1. For an excellent collection of essays on genetic enhancement: E. Parens (ed.), *Enhancing Human Traits: Ethical and Social Implications* (Georgetown University Press, 1998).

Chapter 8

If you want to read more about research in poor countries see Notes and references (above) and also R. Macklin, *Double Standards in Medical Research in Developing Countries* (Cambridge University Press, 2004), written by one of the participants in the CIOMS guidelines. A detailed examination of the ethical issues surrounding consent to participate in medical research is provided in: L. Doyal and J. S. Tobias (eds.), *Informed Consent in Medical Research* (BMJ Books, 2001), pp. 266–76.

There are several guides to the ethical evaluation of medical research that combine some philosophical analysis with practical help for researchers and those on research ethics committees. The most philosophical is D. Evans and M. Evans, *A Decent Proposal: Ethical Review of Clinical Research* (John Wiley & Sons, 1996). For a look at research from goal-based, duty-based and right-based perspectives, and including many case studies, see: C. Foster, *The Ethics of Medical Research on Humans* (Cambridge University Press, 2001).

For a look at the historical background to the control of medical research see: G. J. Annas and M. A. Grodin (eds.), *The Nazi Doctors and the Nuremberg Code: Human Rights in Human Experimentation* (Oxford University Press:, 1992), and for a philosophical overview: B. A. Brody, *The Ethics of Biomedical Research: An International Perspective* (Oxford University Press, 1998).

One important area that I have not even mentioned is the use of animals in medical research. A useful introduction and sourcebook to further reading is: L. Grayson, *Animals in Research: For and Against* (British Library, 2000).

A useful website to guidelines about the ethical conduct of medical research with links to other relevant sites is the UK Department of Health site at: www.corec.org.uk

Index

Index

Visit the
VERY SHORT INTRODUCTIONS
Web site

www.oup.co.uk/vsi

➤ **Information** about all published titles

➤ News of **forthcoming books**

➤ **Extracts** from the books, including titles not yet published

➤ **Reviews** and views

➤ **Links** to other **web sites** and main OUP web page

➤ Information about **VSIs in translation**

➤ **Contact** the editors

➤ **Order** other **VSIs** on-line